MOTHER NATURE
M.D.

ERIC MEYER

FOREWORD BY
JAMES A. DUKE, Ph.D.

PRENTICE HALL
Paramus, New Jersey 07652

Library of Congress Cataloging-in-Publication Data

Meyer, Eric.
    Mother nature, M.D. :protect your health and cure disease with hundreds of healing
foods and herbs / by Eric Meyer.
       p.   cm.
    Includes index.
    ISBN 0-13-032456-6
    1. Naturopathy–Encyclopedias.   2. Herbs–Therapeutic use–Encyclopedias.   3. Dietary
supplements–Encyclopedias.   I. Title.
RZ440 .M476 2001
615.5'35'03—dc21   00-045308
                                                        CIP

Printed in the United States of America

*This book is intended as a reference volume only, not as a medical guide. The information provided is
intended to help the reader make informed decisions about his or her health, but is in no way intended
as a substitute for any professional medical treatments.*

10 9 8 7 6 5 4 3 2

ISBN 0-13-032456-6

ATTENTION: CORPORATIONS AND SCHOOLS

Prentice Hall Books are available at quantity discounts with bulk purchase for educational, business, or sales promotional use. For information, please write to: Prentice Hall Books Special Sales, 240 Frisch Court, Paramus, New Jersey 07652. Please supply: title of book, ISBN, quantity, how the book will be used, date needed.

PRENTICE HALL
Paramus, NJ 07652

http://www.phdirect.com

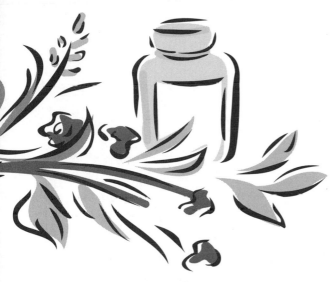

Foreword

Here in my garden in Maryland—a partly-sunny, partly-shaded patch of land I call "The Green Farmacy Garden"—I'm growing many of the very plants that you'll read about in this book. In an area marked "Colds and Flu," I have plenty of onion coming up. In "Cuts and Scrapes," you'll find aloe and goldenseal. My "High Blood Pressure" patch includes a nice stand of garlic. And over in the section labeled "Insomnia," a garden visitor will find lemon balm, camomile, and valerian.

It's no accident that these plants—all, with healing properties—occupy such positions of importance in my Green Farmacy Garden and, also, places of honor in this book. They're all part of what Eric Meyer has called "Mother Nature, M.D."

Of course, one man's pharmacy is not another man's doctor, and each of us has approached the topic of healing plants from different viewpoints. For me, the search for nature's secrets was a long scientific journey, first as a botanist and taxonomist, later as a full-time research scientist for the U.S. Department of Agriculture. In my many years with the USDA I traveled throughout Central America and other parts of the world, discovering, wherever I traveled, traditional healing methods that involved hundreds of common and exotic herbs. Later, my personal explorations led me to develop a comprehensive database, logging in all the known healing effects of thousands of active substances found in plants. (Now that database— "*Father Nature's Farmacy*"—is available to anyone who wants to use it, at *http://www.ars-grin.gov/duke/*.)

In recent years, I'm glad to report that research has confirmed the effectiveness of many healing herbs. Today, scientists are coming to have an even greater understanding of the potent properties of many substances found in living plants. But even so, Mother Nature sometimes works in mysterious ways.

In collecting data about Mother Nature's many healing abilities, Eric Meyer has taken an approach that's not open to experimental scientists— collecting information based on the historical, oral traditions of healing methods as practiced throughout Europe and in parts of the United States. In some cases, the remedies seem homespun, even simplistic. You'll find artichoke for skin problems. Cabbage for quicker healing. Cinnamon for fatigue. But this is no accident. In many homes, these were the remedies that people had on hand for both serious and minor ills. And when these remedies proved effective, the secrets were readily passed along from generation to generation. That's empirical wisdom—and I trust the herbs that are empirically proven more than I trust hastily-approved, new pharmaceuticals.

Science is still at a loss to explain how many of these remedies actually work. But if you've ever put witch hazel on itchy skin, soothed a burn with ice, or eased muscle-ache with a menthol cream, you've already done some experimenting in the vast field of folk remedies. While the sources of this advice were often humble—our own moms, dads, grandparents, and other forebears—the reputation of many of these methods have proven durable.

Often, usefulness is the best test. Just as there is no one remedy that can possibly work for everyone, there are many remedies that may work for some of us. As long as we obey the caution of Hippocrates—"first, do no harm"—we should approach the many traditional forms of healing remedies as an open book.

As I walk through my own Green Farmacy Garden, I often pluck a few leaves here, or take some berries and roots from over there, to treat my own ailments or help out friends and family members. There's no reason why you shouldn't be able to call on *Mother Nature, M.D.,* in the same way.

Obviously, I think Mother Nature is a well-qualified doctor—and quite often, her medicines are better than the best that money can buy in a local pharmacy. I hope this book will help introduce you to her grand, multitudinous, infinitely fascinating, and endlessly resourceful medicine cabinet. My advice: Feel free to take from her ample cornucopia judiciously, and find out what's best for your own health and well-being.

James A. Duke, Ph.D.
Author of *The Green Pharmacy*
and *Dr. Duke's Essential Herbs*

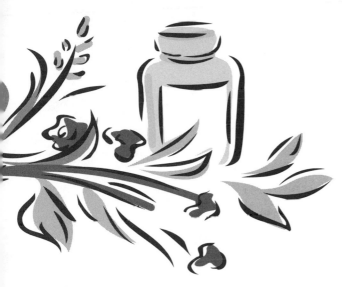

Contents

C

D

E

F

G

H

I

J/K

L

PART I

The Healthy Wonders
of Mother Nature

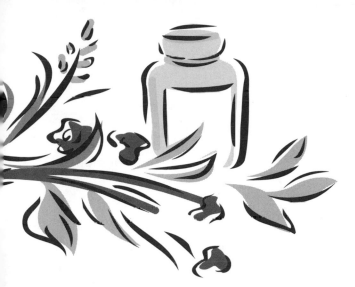

Discovering a Lost World

Since the dawn of time, healers in every culture the world over have studied the healing power of plants. Ancient civilizations from Mesopotamia and China to the Americas and Australia used herbal remedies to treat problems of physical and mental health.

At first, of course, herbal systems were based largely on tradition and folklore, relying on oral transmission from one generation to the next for survival. But over the centuries, the study of the medical botany became increasingly strict and scientifically controlled, gradually moving away from the aura of magic and witchcraft that had often been associated with it in the past.

People began to write down, organize, and categorize their findings. By the eighteenth century, botanical research in Europe had achieved a measure of standardization and coherence that is in keeping with the scientific standards of today. With the advent of the twentieth century, however, the age of Western technology came into full blossom, and the study of medicine took a new direction.

Modern science made huge advances in the fight against infectious disease, turning synthetic antibiotics and antiseptics into the weapons of choice in our medical arsenal. At the same time, medicinal plants were largely forgotten and buried, along with the other follies and superstitions of our ancestors.

HERBS IN WESTERN CIVILIZATION

Most of us know that the countries of Asia have a long tradition of herbalism, but so do those in the West, as history shows.

An Egyptian papyrus dating back to 1700 B.C. mentions the medicinal use of plants, and the ancient Greeks engaged in the systematic study of the curative powers of various botanicals from the time of Pericles (450 B.C.) onward.

An herbal apothecary shop was found in the ruins of Pompeii, which means that herbal medicine was still commonly practiced in the first century A.D. Documents show that extensive research into the medicinal uses of plants was being carried out in monasteries in most parts of Europe up to, and in some cases during, the Middle Ages, when the use of medicinal plants suffered a brief decline. Interest in curative plants revived during the Renaissance. Leonardo da Vinci, aside from his scientific studies and artistic accomplishments, tended an extensive garden of herbs and medicinal plants.

In 1735 Charles de Linné published a classic work of botany, called *The System of Nature*, in which he attempted to classify plants according to flower formation. This book was a benchmark in the scientific study of botany, which went on to reach its zenith in the following century.

A Change of Heart

Our love affair with modern medical technology didn't last, of course. It wasn't long before we began to realize that synthetic medications couldn't cure everything that might go wrong with the human body. There was no "magic bullet." Disorders such as nervous system diseases, coronary diseases, autoimmune diseases, and cancer all proved resistant to conventional treatments.

To make matters worse, we found that if we didn't use our new, synthetic medications wisely, they could actually do more harm than good. They may have been powerful healers, but most came with a host of catastrophic side effects to worry about.

The Times They Are a-Changin'

It's no wonder, then, that recent studies have shown a growing number of people would prefer to go back to natural methods of healing, developed over centuries of practical

THE INDUSTRY OF DISEASE

Although synthetic medicines have proven very effective in treating *acute* illnesses, the medical establishment has yet another strong incentive for prescribing them over natural remedies for *all* conditions: profit.

The manufacture of medicine has become a multibillion-dollar industry that is constantly developing new, more powerful—and more expensive— versions of its products. In fact, fully 50 percent of pharmaceutical medications are replaced every ten years or so. Every year in Canada and the United States, pharmaceutical companies spend about $6,000 per doctor advertising new products. That's a lot of investment. In return, they make a lot of profit.

Here's an example: Over one million people a year develop cancer in the United States alone. Each spends an average of $50,000 a year on treatments, which comes to a total of about fifty billion dollars. And that's just in one country. Experts have even calculated that there are more people who make a living off cancer than there are people who die from the disease!

Obviously, we can't expect multinational pharmaceutical companies to change the situation on their own. They have no reason to. Instead, the change must begin with us, the consumers.

application. The fact that these methods, so often dismissed by the modern medical establishment as nonsense, have proven effective in thousands upon thousands of test cases is ample proof of their value.

After all, even some of our most effective medications—digitalis, quinine, morphine, penicillin, and even aspirin—are derived directly from plants. In fact, 50 percent of our commonly used medications come from botanical sources.

That's not to say that people should ignore the benefits medical science has to offer (and there are many). What we are saying is that, whenever possible, consideration should be given to natural, alternative approaches.

The Synthetic Difference

Even the most sophisticated synthetic products—including those that are derived from plants—don't come close to rivaling the natural complexity of botanicals, and that's an important difference.

OF HORSES, CURES, AND GOVERNMENT SCHIZOPHRENIA

The blame for failing to find a proper role for plant remedies in modern medicine can't all be laid at the feet of the pharmaceutical industry. The government has also contributed its share of confusion to the mix. Here's a case in point.

In 1840, John Hoxsey had to put his best thoroughbred horse out to pasture because of a tumor that had developed on its right leg. As the horse grazed, Hoxsey noticed that it seemed to prefer a particular type of grass over all other available food. Then, after three weeks, he discovered that the tumor had stopped growing. In a year it was cured altogether.

Hoxsey used the plant the horse had been grazing on to concoct a preparation. The recipe has been handed down to various family members, through generations, to the present day. In 1924, John Hoxsey's great grandson set up the first Hoxsey clinic for the treatment of cancer in humans.

Thus began a long and bitter legal battle. Strangely enough, the Hoxsey remedy was never tested by government officials. Doctors argued that taking the cure seriously enough to test it would only bring it to the attention of the public. When Hoxsey was asked to demonstrate the treatment to a group of doctors, he did so without hesitation, and succeeded in curing a patient in an advanced state of illness.

Hoxsey, a miner by profession, eventually agreed to reveal his secret formula, on one condition—that it be made available to anyone, whether they had the means to pay for it or not. He had made a solemn promise to that effect to his father, just before the elder Hoxsey died. For reasons of their own, the doctors to whom he was willing to hand over the formula refused to comply with this condition, and Hoxsey left with his formula intact. The doctors in question denied Hoxsey's version of what took place.

The Hoxsey cure is now banned in the United States, after a legal battle that lasted 35 years! One of the former heads of the operation continues to run a clinic in Tijuana, Mexico, where the treatment is reported to have an 80-percent success rate.

At the same time, New York Botanical Garden recently received a grant of $700,000 from the National Cancer Institute to conduct research on plants that could combat cancer.

Go figure.

When researchers create a new drug, they're not interested in complexity, subtlety, or gentleness, which are the hallmarks of herbal remedies.

Instead, they try to isolate and extract—or synthetically reproduce—single "active ingredients" from plants. This process has given rise to a number of very powerful substances. But it's also what's given rise to the side effects we always see with modern medicines. These can show up as everything from birth defects to cancer.

So there is always a trade-off with modern drugs. They may cure us, but they may also kill us. They are wonderful for treating acute, serious illness very rapidly. Sometimes, that's an option we need. If you're having a heart attack, it's clearly the wrong time to take cholesterol-lowering plant remedies. But if you want to prevent heart attacks or recover from one, then botanicals should be among your considerations.

✍ The Complexity of Plants

The overall effect of a whole-plant remedy—versus the isolated effects of any one of its chemical constituents—is fundamentally different.

The average plant contains between 30 and 150 chemicals. When you drink some herbal tea or a decoction made from a whole plant, a process known as "synergy" takes effect. This means that all the constituents act together to produce the desired effect, and that the same effect cannot be obtained unless *all* the necessary elements are present.

By creating that special kind of balance and allowing many elements to work together to achieve a given result, plant remedies seem to be easier for the body to digest and assimilate and often work without producing harmful side effects.

So, because Mother Nature seems to have provided us with such a fantastic array of medicinal substances, why not make use of them in their original state, as she perhaps intended? It may seem obvious to us, the consumers, but it isn't quite so clear from the perspective of pharmaceutical companies.

✍ Natural Right Versus Copyright

Part of the problem is the way medications are patented. A company that wants to launch a new therapeutic product has to pay for the extensive government-controlled testing that all medications are subjected to. Such testing can commonly cost millions of dollars. Patents, however, can protect only synthetic products, including those derived from plants—but not the plants (or other natural sources) themselves.

Imagine for a moment that you are the CEO of a pharmaceutical company, and you've just spent millions of your company's dollars testing a product made from a plant that anyone could go out and pick for himself from a nearby field. Chances are your stockholders would be somewhat distressed and start looking for a new CEO.

Economic factors force pharmaceutical companies to manufacture and test products that can be protected by patent, and thus remain the exclusive property of the company in question, at least for some years.

This also explains why the medical establishment is vehemently opposed to alternative therapies like homeopathy, acupuncture, osteopathy, plant therapy, and so on, all of which do not rely on synthetic drugs or costly technology to cure patients.

Who, we may ask, benefits most from the system as it now stands—doctors and pharmaceutical companies or patients? There is no doubt that in many instances the use of alternative therapies could alleviate suffering and greatly accelerate the healing process, especially when combined with conventional techniques. And yet, while doctors agree that reducing the amount of medication a patient receives (or eliminating the need for medication altogether) is a good thing, they continue to remain resistant to the idea of using alternative methods of healing.

Fortunately, this attitude is changing, as some enlightened physicians realize that the proper use of alternative methods of healing can benefit both patients and therapists.

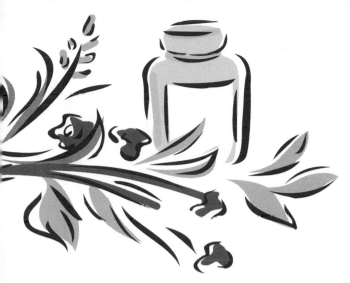

Health and Lifestyle

Doctors who embrace the holistic approach to medicine agree that lifestyle accounts for 70 percent of our state of health. Factors like heredity, biological makeup, medical interventions, and accidents account for the remaining 30 percent.

If they're right, then the conclusion is clear: We can choose whether to be healthy or not. Think of it this way: You are the principal shareholder in your own organism, which means that you hold a controlling interest in your own health capital. The question is, are you going to invest in yourself or not?

✑ Making Wise Investments

The best way to invest in your own future health is to adopt a lifestyle that is appropriate for you. What do we mean by lifestyle? We mean the day-to-day habits that affect your health, such as whether you exercise enough, smoke, eat too much, or drink too much alcohol.

If you're like many people, you don't give lifestyle a second thought. You live from moment to moment, giving into every temptation and appetite, figuring that modern medicine will be equal to the task of fixing anything that might go wrong with you. In other words, you're taking a foolish risk.

It's time you tempered your faith in medical technology with a dose of

AN OLD IDEA WHOSE TIME HAS COME

The idea that disease is caused by organic imbalances is not new. Hippocrates (460–377 B.C.), the father of modern medicine, considered health to be based on a balance of environmental influences, lifestyle, and human characteristics.

Hippocrates also believed that the body possesses its own healing powers, that we are endowed with an innate mechanism designed to maintain or reestablish our inner equilibrium. According to the father of medicine, a doctor's role is, first and foremost, to enhance a patient's natural healing abilities.

reality. You cannot depend on spectacular operations like organ transplants or open-heart surgery to keep you healthy. These interventions are reserved for emergency cases, and are designed to prolong life for a short time. Because the cost of such interventions is extravagant, they're generally reserved for the privileged few. Relying on this kind of technology to revive your health is a little like hoping you'll win the lottery one day.

Let's look at a common, specific example: cancer. We know that the onset of the disease is related to a number of factors, including diet, smoking, and alcohol consumption. A woman's risk of developing breast cancer drops from 1 in 11 to 1 in 24 when her fat intake is reduced from 40 percent to 30 percent of her total diet. That's a reduction of almost 50 percent in her risk of breast cancer, based solely on a change in diet!

Nevertheless, many women go on eating the same fatty foods and hope that a yearly mammogram will keep them safe. If they discover a lump, they'll have it removed.

In other words, they would rather depend on technology to discover the symptoms of an emergency situation—the presence of cancer—than do anything to treat the underlying cause of any potential problem right now.

❧ A State of Balance

The whole idea behind moderating your lifestyle is exactly that: *moderating* it, putting it into a state of balance. And that's where medicinal plants come in.

You start with a problem, a symptom, or malaise, which, if not treated, will eventually result in disease. The symptom can be alleviated, of course, but the important thing is to remove the underlying cause of the problem—or in holistic terms, to restore the body's natural balance. That's what plants do best: restore balance.

Think of the human organism as a precision piece of machinery, like a high-performance car. You know that breakdowns rarely happen out of the blue, that there are always little warning signals beforehand, some noise or feeling that tells you a problem is developing. You also know that one problem often leads to a whole series of other problems.

REESTABLISH YOUR ORGANIC BALANCE

Taking antibiotics to get rid of a minor infection is overkill. It's like using a chain saw to cut a toothpick! But that's not the only problem with them.

As you may know, antibiotics do nothing to strengthen your body's natural immune system. They also have a devastating effect on your intestines, because they destroy beneficial, as well as harmful micro-organisms that grow there. And because harmful bacteria are endowed with their own immune system, they tend to build up a resistance to common types of antibiotics, making them nearly invincible to modern medicine. Relying on less violent remedies when antibiotics are not strictly necessary will help prevent this from happening.

It's up to you to decide whether you want to develop your own immune system, or help bacteria develop theirs!

It's also pretty obvious that it costs less to replace worn parts before a total breakdown occurs, especially when you take factors like towing charges, waiting time, inconvenience, and so on into account. In addition, a serious breakdown—in which the whole automotive system may be thrown out of balance—often causes other damage along with it.

Of course the human body is much more than a simple machine. We have to be wary of comparisons that tend to underestimate the complexity of our organism, the subtle ways in which it reacts, and the delicate state of balance it is able to maintain. However, effective prevention depends on being alert to these early warning signs, in the same way that a mechanic is able to diagnose a major problem from a few minor indications.

HEALTH AND SICKNESS—TWO INSEPARABLE OPPOSITES

Like life and death, light and dark, positive and negative, health and sickness, although opposites, are at the same time united. They form part of the same whole.

So we could say that being healthy implies getting sick from time to time. Your organism is in a state of constant change, as it is forced to adjust to external and internal pressures. Hippocrates defined sickness as an imbalance of the body or mind. Health, on the other hand, can be defined as a state in which balance can be restored fairly quickly, even if it is lost on occasion. Sickness is that state in which the slightest disturbance (a microbe, for example) is capable of throwing our whole system out of balance.

Well-being is therefore a relative state. To remain healthy, an organism must be flexible, in order to adjust to changing circumstances. Lose your flexibility and you lose your health. If your organism can no longer adapt to changing circumstances (and they are always changing), then it becomes increasingly vulnerable to disease. This is exactly what Hippocrates meant when he used the term "dynamic equilibrium" to describe health, over two thousand years ago.

By treating these early warning signs and returning us to balance, botanical remedies represent the best nature has to offer in terms of preventive maintenance.

By contrast, synthetic medications are supposed to be fast-acting, and enable us to get back to our day-to-day activities as soon as possible after an acute and serious health problem.

That's not a bad thing. In fact, in this respect, conventional medicine and a holistic system like plant therapy are perfectly compatible (although some doctors may not agree). So for a complete and well-rounded approach, why not let your doctor take care of fixing the immediate problem, and then use plants to prevent a relapse or another health problem from arising?

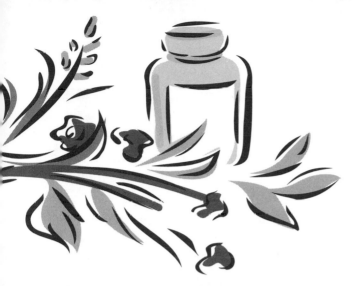

Grow or Buy?

Unless you live in the country, trekking through fields and forests to find fresh medicinal plants, then taking the time to dry and prepare them for use as home remedies may not be a practical option. If you happen to have room in your yard or windowsill for a garden, however, you might want to try growing a few medicinal plants at home. Most of them are not only practical, they're quite beautiful as well.

While it's true that some people claim cultivated herbs are not so effective as herbs gathered in the wild, what counts most, in our opinion, is the quality of care and soil you give your plants. If you grow medicinal herbs in good organic soil and provide plenty of pure water, nutrients, and sunlight, they'll repay your efforts a hundred-fold.

Buying Your Herbs

If you can't grow your own herbs, there's no reason to give up the idea of using herbal remedies. You can now find most locally grown herbs, as well as more exotic varieties, at your local health food or herbal store. And there's an advantage to buying from a herbalist instead of growing or picking your own plants: You'll usually have a wide array of remedies to choose from—including those that are out of season—and often of the highest quality.

Other suppliers, such as pharmacies, generally have personnel on staff who can offer advice about which plant remedies to buy and how to use them. However, you should be aware that there is a big difference between an employee who has a little knowledge about herbal remedies, no matter how well-intentioned he or she may be, and a professionally trained plant therapist.

Here are some suggestions for making sure the herbs you buy are of the very best quality.

Investigate the product. Find out as much as you can about the plants you buy: when and where they were harvested and by whom. Commercially grown plants are generally not so effective as plants that grow in the wild.

See how they're stored. Choose a distributor who stores plants the right way, in order to make sure they lose none of their freshness. Plants should be clearly labeled and kept in opaque containers rather than exposed to sunlight.

Opt for organic. Make sure the plants you use to prepare your medicinal remedies have not been exposed to chemical insecticides or pesticides. A growing number of chemical substances are being used to spray cultivated areas, many of which contain active ingredients that are more toxic than DDT (aldrinine, deildrine, lindane and malathion, to name just a few). In other words, try to obtain only plants that have been grown under organic conditions.

Beware of plastic. Plants packaged in airtight plastic are not guaranteed safe, because fermentation can be a problem.

Look for quality over price. Don't make price your only criterion. It's better to spend a little more on plants that you know are organic than to try to save a few pennies by buying a product that may have been contaminated.

Take a little sniff. Check the odor and appearance of the plants you are buying. If you can smell a plant's natural odor and if it is still green or yellow, then chances are it is fresh. If, on the other hand, a plant's color is dull and gray and if hardly any odor is detectable, then you can suppose it has been lying around for quite some time.

Look for local produce. Opt for plants that grow in the vicinity of your home. The shorter the distance they have been transported, the fresher they are likely to be. Also, some countries systematically spray all agricultural products destined for export, which means that plants may become contaminated with insecticides or pesticides, even though they have been grown under organic conditions.

Find the freshest. In some cases you have to use fresh plants if you want to benefit from their curative properties.

YOUR HERBAL PHARMACY

Once you get your plants home, make sure to store them properly so they'll last as long as possible. The three things you want to watch out for when preserving plants are humidity, light, and air. The best way to store your plants is in sealed, opaque containers, placed in a cool, dark, dry place.

The ideal solution is to have a dry, well-ventilated pantry, sheltered against direct sunlight, that can be used exclusively for storing whole plants and herbal preparations. Make this your personal home pharmacy. Here's how to maintain it:

- Use a separate container for each plant.
- Make sure the containers you use to store plants are thoroughly cleaned and do not retain the odor of previous plants.
- You can store plants in paper or cloth packets or in terra cotta pots, but generally speaking, waterproof opaque glass containers or metal tins (untarnished) are best.
- If you don't have pantry space and intend to keep your plants in the kitchen, make sure your storage containers are opaque.
- As you accumulate more plants, make sure to label all containers clearly (indicating the name of the plant and the date it was harvested) and then arrange them in alphabetical order.
- Spread some fresh lavender around to protect your plants against insects.
- Renew your stock whenever fresh plants become available, because the active ingredients of most plants do not last much longer than a year, even when they are stored properly. Generally speaking, the active ingredients contained in bark and roots last much longer (sometimes for years) than those obtained from leaves and flowers.
- Smell your plants now and then—if they have retained their original odor, they're still in good condition.

Buy whole plants if you can. You can obtain various leaves, roots, shoots, vegetables, and flowers in powdered form, but don't expect them to be fresh. Unscrupulous vendors will even mix one product with another less costly plant in order to increase their profits.

✎ Knowledge That Comes with Experience

No matter how you come by your plants, it's a good idea to get to know some of the types you use most frequently. The more you know about a plant, the better your understanding of its beneficial effects, even if you buy it in capsule form.

Spend some time looking at botanical drawings, visit your local botanical garden, and try to identify various species of plants whenever you take a walk in the countryside. It's exciting to look at a picture of a plant in a book and then find it out in the wild, growing beside a mountain stream, or in a clearing in the woods. In a short time you'll be able to identify a large variety of plants by their color and odor and be familiar with their curative properties. If you can't spend a lot of time outdoors, make it a habit to visit your local herbal store and learn a little more about the more common types of curative plants.

✎ Out in the Wild

If you eventually decide to start gathering your plants from woods and fields, you'll have to make absolutely sure you know what you're picking, so it might be a good idea to check with an herbalist when you first start out, especially if you have any doubts about what a specific type of plant is.

You'll also have to make sure that the plants you gather haven't been sprayed with pesticides or insecticides (remember that aerial spraying of cultivated fields can spread to adjoining areas, as chemical products are diffused by wind) or exposed to other types of pollution. Picking plants that grow near highways, for example, is not a good idea, because they absorb lead emissions from passing cars.

✒ Appreciating Our Natural Treasure

Plants are our friends. They are alive like us. They embellish the planet we cohabit wherever they happen to grow. In this age of scientific progress and accelerated technological development, the world of plants is becoming increasingly vital to our overall well-being, acting as an antidote to the cold urban environment we inhabit, which sometimes seems to be designed more for machines than for people.

Remaining in contact with the botanical world is a way of insulating ourselves against what has come to be called "future shock"—the sense that our rapidly changing world is spinning out of control.

The more knowledge you acquire about plants, the more enthusiastic you'll become about using them, and the more you'll appreciate their beneficial effects. In short, the world of plants will become a part of your life. And the farther you enter into that world, the healthier you will feel.

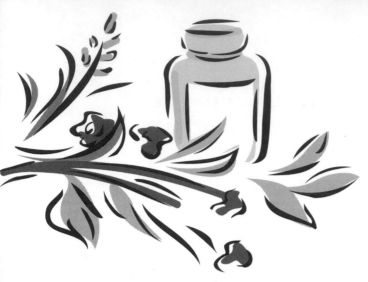

Preparing Your Plant Remedies

Plant remedies come in many forms, and you can make most of them in your own kitchen. The recipes in this book are all chosen for their simplicity and ease of use.

It's generally wiser to prepare one remedy at a time, unless you have a lot of experience. Becoming distracted and making mistakes is too easy otherwise, and you don't want that happening when your health is at stake.

Now, before proceeding to individual remedies, have a look at the detailed instructions below. They'll tell you all you need to know about the various ways of preparing the botanicals you keep in your home herbal pharmacy.

Infusions

It's best to prepare fresh infusions every day. First warm up your teapot with some boiling water. Empty it out, then place the amount of the plant you want to infuse into the pot and pour the indicated amount of boiling water over it. Cover the brew, remove it from the heat, and let it stand for 5 to 15 minutes, depending on the type of plant. Generally speaking, infusions made from leaves or roots should be left standing longer than those made from flowers. In addition, fresh plants tend to infuse much more rapidly than dried plants—only one or two minutes are required.

HERBAL HINT: BULK OR PACKAGED?

Herbal infusions are commonly sold in teabag form; in many cases they are not so effective as infusions made from fresh plants. Drying and shredding plants may be practical for purposes of storage and preparation, but the process also reduces the strength of their active ingredients.

If your only interest is to enjoy a pleasant-tasting beverage, then there is no harm in using teabags, especially because infusions made with fresh plants often have a blander taste. But if you want to take advantage of the medicinal properties of plants like chamomile, mint, linden, and others, try to use fresh ingredients.

The best way to buy herbal products, whether you are looking for leaves, flowers, seeds, or stems, is in bulk form. Opt for plants that have not been cut or shredded, because in many cases roots, rhizomes, bark and sometimes leaves are removed.

After the appropriate amount of time has elapsed, filter the liquid and serve.

Note that although infusions are usually made with the more tender parts of plants (leaves, flowers, and certain seeds). Other parts, such as bark, roots, and rhizomes, can be used in powdered form. Nuts, hard seeds, and buds can also be used after they have been crushed or ground.

If you want to store an infusion for some length of time, filter it while it's still hot, and pour it into an airtight glass container that can be hermetically sealed. You can seal bottles yourself using a cork with a small hole pierced in it. As soon as the cork is in place, seal up the hole with some hot wax.

☙ Decoctions

Bring the required volume of water to a boil, then add the correct amount of the plant you want to use and continue boiling it over low heat for 3 to 30 minutes, as indicated. Let the brew stand for a few minutes, then filter it while it's still hot.

This preparation is used to extract the active ingredients of harder, denser plants, or parts of plants like bark, stems, roots, and so on. Some plants will release their medicinal ingredients only after simmering in boil-

HERBAL HINT: CHOOSING YOUR INSTRUMENTS

Take the time to choose the containers and instruments you use to store plants and prepare your remedies carefully. Here are some tips:

Avoid copper. Don't use copper pots, pot covers, spoons, or containers, because heated copper destroys Vitamin C. Also avoid aluminum. Opt for appliances and instruments made from ceramic or stainless steel whenever possible.

Use a separate pot. It's best to have a teapot that you use exclusively for herbal infusions. Porcelain, glazed pottery, or glass are best.

Strain with fabric. Use a nylon or cotton strainer instead of a metal one.

Work with wood. In some cases it's best to use wooden utensils rather than metal ones (for example, when working with plants that contain tannin).

ing water (over low heat) for a long period of time. Decoctions can be stored in the same way as infusions.

✧ Macerations

Maceration is a process of transforming various parts of a plant into pulp. Plants are soaked in liquid—water, alcohol, or wine—for a few hours. In some cases we recommend steam heating the maceration before drinking it. Don't let plants soak in water for more than twelve hours, to avoid the risk of stagnation.

This process is used to prepare mucilaginous plants or seeds (those that contain thick juices) whose active substances are destroyed when exposed to high temperatures.

✧ Tinctures

A tincture is a form of maceration that uses alcohol instead of water to extract a plant's active ingredient. The main advantage of this type of preparation is that it can be conserved for a long time.

Plants are generally soaked in pure alcohol at temperatures from 120 to 160 degrees Fahrenheit, for one or two weeks. The container should be agitated at least once a day. After the prescribed time period, the alcohol is filtered (in some cases the liquid is repeatedly strained through a coffee filter) and conserved in a cold location.

Use the best quality alcohol you can find (45 to 90 proof) or a clear alcoholic beverage such as vodka, white rum, or eau de vie. Doses are much smaller than infusions: between 5 and 15 drops of tincture as opposed to an entire cup of herbal tea. Drops of tincture can also be added to infusions of the same plant.

HERBAL HINT: THE RIGHT KIND OF WATER

A lot of people are not careful enough about the kind of water they drink. It's always best to use pure spring water when preparing infusions and other herbal remedies. Choose water with a low mineral content, because alkaline water hardens plants and renders their active ingredients less effective.

≈ Medicinal Wine

Wine can also be used to extract the active ingredients of certain plants, although this type of preparation cannot be conserved so long as a tincture. Madeira makes an excellent medicinal wine base. Plants are soaked in the wine for about six days (make sure to agitate the container at least once a day).

≈ Oils

The active ingredients of certain plants are not soluble in water; for these, oil can be used instead. Fill a glass container with plant leaves (don't pack them too tightly) and pour enough extra virgin olive oil to cover them completely. Seal the container and let it stand in direct sunlight or close to some other heat source (at about 70 degrees Fahrenheit) for ten to fifteen days.

≈ Juice and Sap

This preparation consists of extracting the juice or sap of a plant directly. It's an excellent method for applying to vegetables like carrots or celery as well as for certain fleshy medicinal plants. Start by putting the plant through a blender or an extractor, or turning it into pulp by hand, using a porcelain mortar and pestle. Place the pulp in a very fine piece of white cotton gauze and squeeze out the juice or sap. You have to consume the freshly squeezed juice or sap on the same day, unless you refrigerate or deep-freeze it in a hermetically sealed container.

Ointments

Ointments are used for local applications. Like oils, they can be stored for long periods, so you can always have some on hand. Put the flowers, leaves, or stems of the plant (fresh whenever possible) through a blender or extractor or a mortar and pestle. Mix the pulp with lard that has been melted at the lowest possible temperature (never more than 212 degrees Fahrenheit). If you're a vegetarian and object to the use of lard, substitute a vegetable-based product, such as vegetable oil. Remove it from the heat, strain it through a piece of cheesecloth, then let it stand for a day. Strain it a second time through a piece of fine white cotton gauze, and store it in sterile containers.

Poultices

This preparation is designed for local applications of fresh medicinal plants. Put the leaves (or other parts) of the plant in a steamer, over a pot of boiling water. When the leaves are hot and soft, lay them out on some fine material (cotton or linen is best). Layer leaves and material for increased thickness. When the poultice is cool enough, apply directly to the affected area.

You can also grind the plant in a blender or with a mortar and pestle, and then spread it on the material. For best results, these poultices should be applied as soon as possible after grinding (except for certain plants like aloe vera, which require special preparations).

Compresses

Soak some clean white cotton in a hot infusion or decoction, squeeze it out, and apply it to the affected area.

You can also apply material that has been soaked in an infusion, decoction, or medicinal oil without squeezing it out. Compresses are generally applied to healthy skin, where there is no risk of infection. If a skin eruption is likely to turn into an abscess or open sore, do not apply a compress.

☙ Essential Oils

Essential oils are practical and relatively easy to prepare. Crush a plant in a mortar and pestle until you end up with a paste. Place in an appropriately sized container and cover with pure vegetable oil (sweet almond or corn oil, for example). Add a teaspoon of cider vinegar and seal the container so that it is airtight. Don't fill the container right up to the top, as you will have to agitate the liquid regularly. Place it in direct sunlight or near a heat source and let it stand for one month. Strain the mixture through fine cotton or cheesecloth, pressing as much of the oil through as you can. If the essential oil doesn't seem strong enough, repeat the process with the same oil and some fresh plant.

Note that these essential oils are for external use only. Those that can be used internally are always labeled "for medicinal purposes" and require a more sophisticated method of preparation.

☙ Essences

Dilute a small amount (about one-third of a fluid ounce) of essential oil in one quart of alcohol or vinegar and use the mixture as a skin freshener. You can prepare wonderful smelling essences using your favorite scented plants: lavender, eucalyptus, rosemary, mint, or rose.

HERBAL HINT: WORKING WITH TASTE

Anything that isn't sweet tastes bitter or sour. But by sweetening everything you eat or drink, you deprive yourself of the wide range of taste sensations the world of plants has to offer. In fact, plants are just as varied in taste as they are in color or size.

Try not to sweeten your herbal infusions all the time. If you really don't like the taste of a certain herb, add a zest of lemon. And if you have to use a sweetener, opt for pure, natural honey.

HERBAL HINT: TAKING THE RIGHT DOSAGES

Recommended dosages are generally based on average requirements. Use your judgment to make adjustments according to size, weight, or age. For example, a healthy young man, six feet tall, and weighing 190 pounds should receive a considerably stronger dose than a rather frail, elderly person, weighing 120 pounds. For children, cut recommended dosages in half.

Remember to spread doses throughout the day. For example, the usual recommended dosage for herbal infusions is three to six cups per day. But don't drink them all at once. Drink half a cup to a cup of infusion three times a day before meals.

Once you've started on a remedy, give it a little time to work. Observe how your body reacts to a given treatment. Generally speaking, if you don't see any positive results in three or four days, you may want to stop the treatment and try something else.

❧ Inhalations

Prepare an infusion in a large pot. Using a towel to cover your head, lean over the pot, and inhale the rising steam. This technique is excellent for decongesting respiratory passages, as well as opening clogged pores of the skin.

❧ Fumigation

This technique consists of boiling a plant in a sickroom, in order to fill the room with a particular herbal odor.

❧ Baths

Add four or five quarts of an infusion, decoction, or maceration to your bath water. For best results, the bath water should be maintained at about 100 degrees Fahrenheit, and you should remain in the bath for about 20 minutes. Wrap yourself in a towel or terry cloth bathrobe afterwards, and lie down for an hour.

✑ Other Methods

Other preparations include syrups, unguents, suppositories, enemas, lotions (usually cooled infusions spread on the body), drops (especially for the eyes and ears), gargles, vaginal douches, sitz baths, and capsules made from dried powder.

PART II

The Healing Powers
of Nature's Medicinals

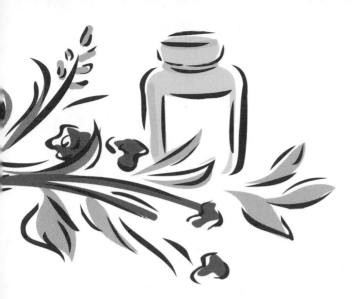

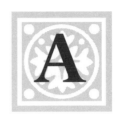

✎ Abscesses

So much pain for such a small problem. Whether you call them common boils or abscesses, they're among the most uncomfortable infections you can get, and antibiotics don't help.

Abscesses are easy to recognize; they're accumulations of pus that form under the skin. Often, they're inflamed—the affected area becomes red and painful to the touch—and sometimes they even cause a slight fever.

Unfortunately, they're devilishly difficult to prevent, because so many things can cause them. You can get boils from having too much oil in the skin, from ingrown hairs, from sitting too long in one place, from splinters, and from a dozen other causes. Any time there's an opening in the skin where bacteria can enter, you're at risk for getting an abscess. With proper treatment, however, you can heal these painful annoyances quickly and safely.

Heed the Signs

Although abscesses are relatively minor disorders, don't make the mistake of neglecting them. A condition called *erysipelas* is characterized by the appearance of a number of abscesses at the same time. Chronic abscesses are often tubercular infections. Likewise, if you're fighting a chronic illness, such as cancer, diabetes, or rheumatoid arthritis, or you're taking an anti-inflammatory drug, such as Prednisone, a boil can become dangerous. For any of these conditions, you'll need the help of a health care professional.

Also, abscesses that occur deep inside the body, in the liver, lungs, kidneys, and even the brain, for example, can be extremely dangerous and require professional medical attention, as can those that occur between the crack of the buttocks (pylonidal cysts).

Remedy the Situation

For small, common boils, home treatment is your best option. An abscess has to drain before it can heal, but trying to drain it before it's "ripe" won't do much good. Generally, you'll have to wait until the skin over the infection softens and comes to a small, white "head." Then the application of some moist heat will encourage it to open on its own. If the abscess opens and drains spontaneously, clean the wound, then dress it with a sterile gauze. If the abscess is a large one and doesn't open, it may need to be lanced. This should be done by a health care professional.

Plant Power

Here are some remedies that can help encourage spontaneous draining and speed your recovery.

Ladies mantle can be used in a poultice. Rinse some leaves (enough to cover the affected area), crush them into a pulp, and apply them locally.

Burdock can be prepared as an infusion or concentrated decoction that helps prevent secondary infections. For local applications, use pulp made from cooked roots and young leaves. To prepare a concentrated decoction, boil 60 to 100 grams in one liter of water for about 15 minutes.

Cow parsnip is a treatment for abscesses that are not inflamed. Apply crushed fresh leaves and roots to the affected area.

Birch buds can be made into a decoction that can help soothe pain. Use 30 grams of birch buds in a liter of water and drink four or five cups during the course of the day.

Cabbage may be a common vegetable, but it can also be used to make effective compresses. Take some fresh, washed leaves, cut away the edges, place them between two pieces of clean cotton, and heat them briefly with a hot iron. Then apply them directly to the skin. You can also soak your cabbage leaves in hot water and apply them to the skin, changing the leaves frequently.

Marshmallow is an herb that can be used both externally (as a compress) and internally: Drink two cups of decoction a day, made from marshmallow flowers (30 grams in a liter of water). For a compress, soak the leaves in very warm water and lay them gently over the affected area.

≈ Acne

Acne is generally the result of hyperactive sebaceous glands, which are a side effect of the hormonal surges that occur during adolescence. It is also a bane and a curse that can make people feel so unsightly that they have been known to lock themselves away and refuse to make public appearances during a breakout. For young people, the scars acne leaves can be both physical and emotional. But there are a number of measures you can take to control the problem and prevent permanent damage to the skin.

A TREAT FOR THE FEET AND MORE

Malva, also known as musk mallow, is an unusual herb with a very specialized use: treating abscesses on the hands or feet. Soak two handfuls of flowers in five liters of cold water overnight. Next day heat the water and soak the affected area for 20 minutes at a time. The same leaves can be applied locally: Heat them up in a little water, add some barley flour to thicken, then spread the mix on a piece of cotton or linen and apply it, still warm, to the affected area.

The uses of malva don't end at the extremities. You can also make an infusion from the dried plant (1 oz of herb to 1 oz of water) that acts as a cough syrup.

And for sheer culinary pleasure, try dressing up a salad with its pretty pink and white flowers, or create a side dish by boiling the roots and leaves. Malva is chock full of vitamins A, B, and C, so you can't go wrong by adding it to a meal.

You can find malva at specialty shops or order it by mail over the Internet.

Basic Skin Care

Keep your skin clean, using a mild soap or an astringent cleansing product specially designed for oily skin, but don't overdo it. Scrubbing too much can stimulate sebaceous glands to produce even more oil and can actually make the problem worse.

BLACKHEADS AND HOW THEY GET THAT WAY

Why are blackheads black? Well, the reason is oxidation: Sebum, secreted by pores, is composed of fat, which oxidizes when it comes in contact with the air. That is why persons with greasy skin are more likely to develop blackheads which, if left unattended, cause acne pimples.

If you have greasy skin it may be necessary to modify your diet in order to eliminate excess fats and sugars.

Don't squeeze blackheads without cleaning and preparing your skin first. The last thing you want to do is develop infections, which can leave deep scars in your skin.

First clean your skin and hands with a mild antiseptic soap. Then rub a slice of tomato or lemon on the area of skin you intend to clean. Lemon especially has an astringent effect. Use it pure or mixed with a little rose water. After you remove your blackheads, make sure to keep your skin as clean and free of grease as possible, in order to prevent further accumulations of sebum from blocking pores.

Here are some other plants that can help eliminate blackheads from your life:

Celandine makes an effective treatment for a number of skin problems, including warts, corns, and calluses. Mix celandine with couchgrass to treat blackheads: Soak five grams of fresh celandine leaves and flowers and five grams of couchgrass in a liter of spring water for a few hours; dip some sterile gauze or cotton in the liquid to make compresses, and apply directly to affected areas.

Bedstraw is another effective treatment for blackheads. Wash the plant and use an extractor to make fresh juice, which you apply immediately to affected areas of skin.

If you are no longer an adolescent and still suffer from acne (so-called "juvenile" acne sometimes persists up to the age of 35) your best bet is to rely on plants like ginseng and gotu-kola, both of which help your body adapt to stress.

Eating Well

Good nutrition is as important as skin hygiene when it comes to beating acne. Here are some strategies you can use to keep your complexion clear and attractive.

Take the salt off the table. Reduce your salt intake as much as possible. High salt intake seems to cause acne flare ups.

Avoid iodine. Although a small amount of iodine is necessary for good health, too much can stir up acne. Common table salt, shellfish, and spices are all sources of iodine.

Eliminate sweets. Although chocolate has long been branded the bad guy where acne is concerned, it's not the cocoa but the sugar that causes the problem. Avoid chocolate, of course, but also steer clear of anything else made from white sugar or refined flour.

Ban beef and pork. Fatty foods will play havoc with your skin. Leave beef, pork, nuts, and cheese on the shelves of the grocery store.

Eat from the garden. Consume as many raw vegetables and fruits as you like, especially those that contain high levels of Vitamins A (wheat, chard, raw carrot, celery, cherry, cabbage, cauliflower, squash, watercress, endive, spinach, virgin vegetable oils, lettuce, corn, mandarins, olive, oranges, barley, nettle, sorrel, parsley, green pepper, dandelion, fresh peas, plums, prunes, escarole, tomato, and sunflower), vitamin D (fish oils), and biotin (bananas, wheat, mushrooms, spinach, green beans, brewer's yeast, corn, bee pollen, potatoes, whole grain rice, and tomatoes).

Liquefy. Drink as much pure spring water as you can, and have two glasses of watercress and orange juice, mixed in equal parts, every day.

Internal Applications

Artichoke is recommended for cases of acne related to a liver or kidney problem. Prepare infusions using leaves and roots: 30 grams of leaves in a liter of water. Drink three cups a day, sweetened with honey to mask the plant's bitter taste. Or prepare a tincture: Cut and dry your own artichoke leaves, then soak 500 grams in distilled spirits (vodka or brandy) for 15 days; press, extracting as much liquid as you can from the leaves; take one or two teaspoons before meals.

Burdock is one of the best remedies for acne because of its antiseptic properties. Infuse 50 to 60 grams of fresh roots in a liter of water and drink three to five cups a day. You can also prepare an extraction, using 50 grams to a liter of water.

Asian ginseng is recommended for persons who are past adolescence, or who have tried other plant remedies without success. You can buy dried Asian ginseng roots in most health food stores. Younger, more active persons should not take ginseng for more than three weeks at a time. To prepare an infusion, use two or three grams per cup of boiling water and let the brew stand for 10 minutes. If you take liquid ginseng extract (in vial or capsule form), take one vial or capsule a day for 10 days, and then stop. Repeat every two months or so.

Wild pansy is a flower remedy recommended for persons suffering from juvenile acne. Boil 20 grams of dried plant in a liter of water for 10 minutes and drink four or five cups a day.

Sage is a common cooking herb that can also be used to make lotions or compresses. Local applications of sage help maintain healthy skin and combat the formation of pimples.

External Applications

Burdock makes a great ointment that you can use for local applications. Crush some fresh leaves in a mortar and pestle, then soak them in a little olive oil, in a sealed container, for 24 hours (place the container in a warm location). Filter out the leaves and apply the oil to skin that's broken out with acne (the preparation will remain active for a few days).

PERSONALIZE YOUR ANTI-ANEMIA DIET

Different people have different needs and tastes, depending upon their age, situation, and gender. Look for the category that best describes you and choose from the foods that best suit your needs.

Pregnant women: broccoli, plums, haddock, spinach.
Breast-feeding women: turkey (dark meat), raw spinach, dried apricots, potatoes.
Infants: barley, oat and rice cereal, fruit juice.
Children: lean beef, turkey (white meat), almonds, oranges.
Teenage boys: beef, turkey (dark meat), almonds, oranges.
Teenage girls: grapes, sunflower seeds, dried apricots, grapefruit juice.
Elderly persons: turkey (white meat), plums or prunes, tomato juice.
Active women: lima beans, soy beans, grapes, orange juice.
Active men: Soy beans, molasses, hamburger meat (pure beef), orange juice.

For cases of follicular acne, prepare a paste using crushed burdock roots; apply the paste, and leave it in place for about half an hour.

Celery masks make an effective acne remedy, believe it or not. Crush some celery in a mortar and pestle, apply locally and leave in place for about half an hour; remove the mask by rubbing it gently with some unflavored yogurt.

Fresh cabbage juice, put into compresses or lotions, is excellent when combined with internal applications of cabbage decoction (15 grams boiled milk) taken morning and night.

Bedstraw ointment can be made into an effective lotion. Mix some of the plant's fresh juice with a little butter at room temperature and apply it to the skin.

Tomato and sorrel work well together to fight acne. First place a slice of tomato on the skin; half an hour later remove the tomato (don't wash your skin) and apply some freshly crushed sorrel leaves; leave in place for another half hour, then rinse with fresh water.

≈ Anemia

The poet Sir John Suckling once opined, "Why so pale and wan, fond lover? Prithee, why so pale and wan?" The prosaic answer, unfortunately, might have been, "Not enough iron in my diet. I'm becoming a little anemic."

A very pale complexion is a common symptom of anemia, as are listlessness, physical and mental fatigue, and sometimes dizziness, fainting spells, and palpitations. A blood test is usually required in order to obtain an accurate diagnosis of anemia.

The condition generally results from lack of red blood corpuscles (or hemoglobin) in the blood. Your body needs iron to produce hemoglobin, which carries oxygen to tissues and cells. When you don't take in enough iron, you don't make enough hemoglobin. Women are more likely to develop anemia, because of blood loss and a resulting iron deficiency during menstruation.

DO COPPER BRACELETS REALLY WORK?

As an essential mineral, we need copper in our diets. It helps protect against anemia, and it even may help defend us from the effects of environmental pollutants. But wearing copper?

According to legend, copper jewelry—usually in the form of a bracelet—helps to ease the pain of arthritis. It sounds like quackery, but there may be something to it. A double-blind study in Australia concluded that copper bracelets actually do reduce pain and inflammation.

How could that be? Theoretically, copper is absorbed through the skin and binds with another compound in the system that together act as an anti-inflammatory. Copper is also an antioxidant and may in that way help in the treatment of arthritis.

Good sources of copper include many members of the nut family, including peanuts, Brazil nuts, walnuts, hazelnuts, almonds, and pecans; as well as sunflower oil and buckwheat.

Nutrition

Make sure your diet is varied and rich in iron-containing foods. These include liver (150 to 200 grams, boiled or grilled over low heat every day), lima beans, sunflower seeds, dried apricots, raw broccoli, spinach, almonds, sweet peas, and poultry. At the same time, don't overload your digestive system by eating too much. Moderation is the key.

Here are some dietary tips to help you keep your iron levels up to par.

Make a veggie cocktail. Drink a quarter cup of beet juice, mixed with an equal amount of fresh carrot juice, every day. This will help to re-mineralize your body in general.

Have some honey, honey. Honey, which helps your body assimilate calcium, is also useful for combating anemia. Use the purest honey you can find, generally available in herbal and health food stores, or directly from a beekeeper.

Get your three B's. Look for foods that contain Vitamins B1 (garlic, apricots, algae, peanuts, oats, bananas, wheat, wheat germ, blackcurrant, cabbage, dates, dried figs, sprouted wheat, dried beans, lentils, brewer's yeast, melon, hazelnuts, walnuts, barley, oranges, whole grain bread, parsley, dried peas, apples, plums, raisins, lettuce, buckwheat, and soy); B9, better known as folic acid (asparagus, carrots, spinach, and wheat germ); and B12 (algae and pollen). B12 is especially important for keeping anemia at bay. Fresh brewer's yeast contains all three of these essential vitamins.

Plant Power

In addition to the dietary changes mentioned above, you can combat anemia by using the herbs mentioned below.

Elecampane is especially recommended for younger women. Make a decoction by adding 20 to 40 grams of freshly crushed roots to a liter of cold water; boil for one minute, then let stand for 10 minutes; drink a cup before meals (sweeten with a little honey if you find the bitter taste too pronounced).

Centaury is a pretty purple flower that makes an excellent general tonic, although it should not be used over extended periods of time because it tends to irritate mucous membranes lining the gastrointestinal tract. Because centaury infusions taste bitter, mix 10 grams of the plant with 10 grams of absinthe and 10 grams of buckbean, add to one liter of sweet wine and let stand for some hours; filter and drink one wine glass before meals.

Blessed thistle is excellent for stimulating your appetite. Taken as an infusion, it helps combat anemia. Add 30 to 50 grams to a liter of boiling water, let stand for 10 minutes, and drink three cups a day.

Ash makes a beneficial tonic, which should be used prudently. Drink two or three cups of ash infusion a day, between meals. Use 20 to 30 grams of leaves in a liter of boiling water, and let stand for 10 minutes.

Fenugreek stimulates your overall metabolism and helps restore your appetite. Eat two teaspoons a day, mixed with honey, and spread on some spiced bread or chocolate. Or you can prepare a decoction: Boil a handful of coarsely ground seeds in a liter of water for a few minutes, then let stand for 10 minutes.

Gentian is also great for stimulating appetite. An infusion of the roots of this beautiful flower can be used as an aperitif before meals, and as a digestive after eating. Pour a cup of boiling water over three grams of roots, and let stand for an hour.

Hops is an essential ingredient in beer brewing and—not surprisingly—

has a calming effect on the nervous system; it also makes an excellent tonic for persons suffering from anemia and fatigue. Hops infusions help regenerate the blood: Add 20 to 30 grams of cones to a liter of boiling water, and let stand for 10 minutes. Use honey to neutralize the bitter taste.

Buck bean (bog bean) makes a tonic that stimulates appetite and digestion, and is especially recommended for nervous persons. Prepare infusions using a tablespoon of shredded plant to a cup of boiling water, and drink with meals. You can also obtain buck bean in powdered form: Take two or three grams a day.

Nettle is rich in calcium, phosphorous, and other minerals, as well as Vitamin D, so it makes an excellent treatment for anemia. You can buy fresh nettle extract (brand name—Urtica Primera) or prepare nettle infusions: Use one heaping teaspoon in a quarter of a liter of water, let stand for 10 minutes, and drink before meals. For severe cases of anemia, you can drink up to two liters a day. You can also add nettles to salads.

❧ Anxiety

It's like spending every hour of every day balancing on a high wire between two skyscrapers and never knowing when a sudden gust of wind might give you a little nudge. The emotional tension of chronic anxiety can be totally debilitating. It makes people tense and unproductive and often destroys their relations with friends and family. It even causes physical symptoms, such as trembling, shortness of breath, accelerated heartbeat, palpitations, and a feeling of suffocation.

Because anxiety does, so often, manifest itself in the form of physical symptoms, a treatment based on a physical approach can be of great benefit and may ultimately solve the psychological aspects of the problem as well.

Lifestyle

Ask yourself, what exactly makes you anxious? Perhaps the problems in your life seem insurmountable right now. Consider them as a message telling you to take a good hard look at your life. Do you have habits that need changing? Beliefs that need to be revised? If you're sincere in your desire to turn your life around and positive in your approach, you will succeed.

Also take a close look at any habits you may have that are harmful to your health. Although such habits (such as using drugs or alcohol) may help you get through a difficult day, they're not true friends. Even socially acceptable habits like smoking or drinking coffee or tea will have a detrimental effect on both your physical health and state of mind over the long term.

Here are some other tips that can help you tame the anxiety monster.

Plan your time with your health in mind. It's a good idea for persons suffering from anxiety to organize their day-to-day activities as much as possible. Setting aside some time for relaxation and meditation is especially important.

Go to a pro. Psychotherapy has become more accessible in recent years and offers a number of preventive techniques. But not all therapists offer the same product. If you go to a psychiatrist— that is, a medical doctor with some training in treating psychiatric disorders—he may recommend medication. Our advice: Try to avoid taking tranquilizers. Although they may help alleviate feelings of anxiety momentarily, they are really only a way of avoiding problems that have to be confronted sooner or later. Psychologists, social workers, and other lay therapists are more likely to do some form of "talking" therapy.

Take a walk in the woods. Get out and enjoy the beauty and tranquillity of nature as often as you can. Reestablishing contact with the source of life can do wonders for your state of mind.

Nutrition

Research conducted in the United States has shown that young persons convicted of committing delinquent acts tend to eat excessive amounts of sweets of all kinds. When the amount of sugar in their diet is reduced— which turns out to be a very difficult thing to do because they seem to crave sugar so much—their behavior becomes significantly less aggressive.

Obviously, what we eat in our daily diet can exert an effect on our psychology. So can certain plants, when used medicinally—it's up to us to take advantage of their potential benefits—in conjunction with more conventional forms of therapy. There is no doubt that certain conventional medications have helped large numbers of anxious or depressed people regain a measure of mental stability, allowing them to lead relatively normal lives.

Try to adhere to a diet rich in vitamins and minerals. Brewer's yeast, which contains most of the B-complex vitamins as well as Vitamin D, is especially recommended. Eat a healthy balanced diet of nonrefined, non-processed foods, as free as possible of contaminants like pesticides, insecticides, chemical fertilizers, and so on.

Plant Power

As far as plants are concerned, the simple act of preparing an infusion can often soothe the mind and dispel unfounded fears. Handling plants is a good way to "return to your roots" so to speak, and regain a sense of inner peace and harmony. Here are some suggestions.

Hawthorn is a plant of choice for the treatment of anxiety, and should be one of the first remedies you try. Use a teaspoon of flowers in a cup of boiling water, and drink three or four cups a day.

Basil is a common cooking herb and a natural sedative that helps alleviate anxiety, insomnia, and other nervous disorders. To prepare your infusions, which you should drink after meals and before going to bed, drop a few pinches of fresh or dried basil in a cup of boiled water, stir, and filter.

Lavender is a lovely wild flower that helps alleviate symptoms like trembling, general agitation, and nervousness. Use an extraction: Boil 20 or 30 grams of lavender in a liter of water for a few minutes, then let stand for half an hour, filter, and drink.

Lemon balm (melissa) is known to alleviate nervousness. Melissa is especially recommended for women suffering from anxiety during menstrual periods. Use 20 to 30 grams to a liter of boiling water, and infuse for 10 minutes. Drink two or three cups a day.

Orange flowers can help persons suffering from nervousness, anxiety, insomnia, migraines, and even hysteria. It's a good idea to keep some orange flower water at home, in case a crisis situation arises. You can also prepare infusions using 25 grams of flowers to a liter of boiling water.

Linden tree flower is a well-known sedative that gently soothes the nervous system. It is most effective for the treatment of general agitation or fatigue caused by fragile nerves or overwork, especially when the condition results in digestive problems. Add about 25 grams of flowers to a liter of boiling water and let stand for 10 minutes. Linden baths can be effective for calming agitated children: Simply add a linden decoction (boil 500 grams of flowers and leaves in two liters of water for 25 minutes, then filter) to your child's bath water.

Valerian is a powerful sedative and antispasmodic and is very useful for alleviating excitability and agitation caused by anxiety. It will also help you sleep if you can't manage to stop your thoughts from keeping you awake. Use the dried root to prepare a decoction: Add between 30 and 60 grams (depending on how strong you want the effect to be) to a liter of water, boil for a few minutes, and then let stand for 10 minutes. For cases of insomnia, add some linden flowers. Valerian has a very pungent odor. For this reason, many people prefer taking it in capsule form.

❧ Appetite Problems

Losing your appetite is a little like losing your desire to live. The cause may have nothing to do with food. Instead it may be linked to some profound sense of dissatisfaction, some existential "angst," or to a more general physical problem. It is normal, for example, to eat less when you are sick; the body, in order to give itself a chance to eliminate toxins, tends to crave less food when something goes wrong.

If, however, your lack of appetite is not related to an illness, you should take appropriate steps to remedy the situation.

Lifestyle

Your state of mind can affect both your appetite and your digestion. Here are some tips for keeping both in tiptop shape.

Avoid controversy. Stay away from touchy subjects and confrontational situations at the dinner table. Instead, try to fully enjoy the food and company you have been blessed with, and drink some mint or orange tea to calm your passions if someone else happens to start an argument.

Create a pleasant atmosphere. Atmosphere can make all the difference, especially during periods of stress—for example, when you are under a lot of pressure at work. Try candles or quiet background music. And don't be in a rush to get through the meal.

Do some culinary design. You want the meals you serve to taste terrific, of course, but you should also try to make them look as attractive as possible. Food that looks appealing also stimulates your appetite.

Nutrition

The plant world offers a wide variety of cures for problems ranging from a temporary lack of appetite due to mild depression to conditions like anorexia. Certain vegetables, spices, condiments, and aromatic herbs are remarkably effective for stimulating appetite and should become a regular part of your diet. These include alfalfa sprouts, artichokes, celery, parsley, onions, watercress, black radish, leeks, cardamom, cayenne, chicory, garlic, fennel, juniper, mint, horseradish, rosemary, savory, marjoram, gooseberries, sage, wild thyme, thyme, and verbena.

Plant Power

Here are some other herbs that are great for stimulating a flagging appetite.

Absinthe is very beneficial for the stomach. In addition to stimulating appetite, it alleviates gastric pain, nausea, heartburn, and flatulence. It also stimulates liver function and improves blood circulation. Prepare infusions using two or three grams to a cup of water, and drink in small amounts throughout the day. *Important: Breast-feeding mothers should not take absinthe.*

Angelica alleviates flatulence and improves kidney function. It is effective for the treatment of all kinds of stomach problems, including ulcers and vomiting accompanied by cramps. Prepare infusions using a teaspoon of ground seeds to a half cup of boiled water.

Aniseed is an aromatic plant that helps digestion, stimulates appetite, and acts as a general tonic for the stomach. It is recommended for persons whose appetite loss is related to overwork and who suffer from stomach cramps or spasms. You can buy anisette, a well-known digestive beverage, or prepare aniseed infusions: Add a teaspoon of ground seeds to a cup of boiled water, infuse for 10 minutes, and filter. Sip small amounts throughout the course of the day (one cup a day in all).

Elecampane helps digestion, stimulates appetite, and regulates liver functions. It is useful in cases of general fatigue, anemia, and sluggish digestion. Prepare decoctions using 30 to 40 grams of crushed roots per liter of cold water; bring to a boil for one minute, then let stand for 10 to 20 minutes. You can also drink infusions: 20 to 30 grams of roots per liter of boiling water.

Chamomile aids digestion, stimulates appetite, and acts as a mild sedative. If you suffer from difficult digestion, stomach spasms, constipation, or diarrhea, try drinking chamomile infusions a half hour before meals (not after meals, as many people tend to do). Use a teaspoon of Anthemis nobilis flowers (the amount varies depending on which type of chamomile you buy, so check the label on the package or ask your herbalist how much you should use) to a cup of boiled water, and let it stand for half an hour. Drink one cup a day (children should be given half a teaspoon every half hour).

Caraway seeds stimulate sluggish digestive functions and appetite, and help cure colic in young infants. Nervous persons suffering from stomach pain and/or spasms should also use caraway. To prepare infusions, add three teaspoons of ground seeds to a cup of boiled water and let it stand for a few minutes. Drink three cups a day.

Centaury is very effective in cases where loss of appetite is accompanied by painful digestion and intestinal fermentation. It also helps combat anemia, asthenia, and general fatigue; stimulates the salivary glands, stomach, and intestines; and alleviates constipation and flatulence. Depurative herbal tea is recommended for cases of anemia and depression. In addition to stimulating appetite, it has a beneficial effect on kidney function.

Gentian is a common medicinal that is well known for its beneficial effect on the stomach. The plant stimulates appetite and digestive functions, activates the salivary glands, and promotes increased production of white blood cells, which is important in the treatment of anemia and asthenia. Prepare decoctions by soaking a teaspoon of roots in a cup of water for four hours. Drink a teaspoon every two hours, or before meals (at least half an hour before eating to give the plant time to take effect). You should not take gentian for prolonged periods, as the plant can cause mild side effects like headaches or nausea.

Ginseng helps stimulate appetite and restores strength and vigor to organisms suffering from fatigue. To prepare infusions, use about two grams of dried roots to a cup of boiling water and let stand for five to 10 minutes.

Younger, more active persons should not take ginseng for more than three weeks at a time. If you prefer buying commercial ginseng, available in liquid form, don't take more than one vial a day, for a period of 10 days, and repeat the cure every two months or so.

Hops stimulate appetite and reduce flatulence and intestinal spasms. They also have a soothing effect on the nervous system and are recommended for cases of nervous tension and/or diarrhea. Infuse two or three grams of cones in a quarter of a liter of water. Avoid excessive doses or prolonged use.

Horehound not only stimulates appetite, but is also very effective for combating the flu and bronchitis (although you should remember that when you are ill, eating less is a natural reaction, allowing your body to eliminate toxins). Because infusions are so mild, take one or two grams in tablet form, along with your meals.

Sage stimulates appetite and alleviates diarrhea, as well as other intestinal problems. Prepare an infusion using one teaspoon of powdered sage per quarter liter of boiling water; let it stand for five minutes. Sage also helps reduce fever, and is recommended for cases of fatigue and nervous tension. Aperitif herbal tea is recommended for cases of anemia and anorexia: Mix equal amounts of ironweed, centaury, gentian, and vervain; add about a teaspoon and a half of the mixture to a cup of boiling water, and let it stand for five minutes.

❧ Arrhythmia

Arrhythmia is a general term that refers to any situation where the heart does not beat regularly. The condition can have serious consequences, but in most cases, it simply makes the heart less resistant to effort and/or stress.

There are a number of possible causes of arrhythmia, ranging from nervousness to chronic constipation or flatulence, food poisoning, tobacco addiction, spinal cord lesions, and so on. A doctor should be consulted, except for the most benign cases. The remedies listed below are in no way meant to replace medical treatment.

A very slow pulse of between 50 and 60 beats per minute can be the result of an infection, some type of intoxication, difficult convalescence, jaundice, etc.

In addition to the treatment prescribed by your doctor, you should avoid placing any kind of strain on your heart while carrying out your daily activities, and adopt a diet composed of light foods, containing few if any stimulants and very little salt.

If the condition becomes permanent, you may have to spend most of your time in bed. You should, however, do your best to exercise your legs regularly. If they are left completely immobile, you may develop a condition known as thrombosis, characterized by blood coagulating in the veins in your legs.

Lifestyle

If your heartbeat is chronically fast and irregular (paroxystic tachycardia), don't depend solely on medical treatments to remedy the situation. It's up to you to make the necessary changes to your lifestyle that will enable you to slow down and lead a calmer, more relaxed existence. Although not always easy, making these changes is essential if you want to enjoy the fruits of your labors for any length of time.

Nutrition

Do everything you can to avoid stimulants like coffee, tea, alcohol, and tobacco. Cut out salt altogether, adopt a hypotoxic diet, and make sure you ingest a lot of Vitamins B1 and C.

Note: Although plant therapists have traditionally prescribed lily of the valley and digitalis to treat cardiac problems, these plants can be dangerous when taken without medical supervision. Both are used as ingredients for homeopathic remedies and allopathic medications designed to treat heart disorders.

Plant Power

The plants mentioned below are offered only as an adjunct to and not a replacement for your doctor's recommendations. Make certain that you let your doctor know about any herbal remedies you're using.

Hawthorn regulates heart functions. It acts as a stimulant, and at the same time has a calming, beneficial effect on the organism as a whole, affecting both the heart and the nervous system. For that reason it is especially recommended for cases of arrhythmia. To prepare infusions add 1/3 oz of flower tops to a liter of boiling water and let stand for 15 minutes.

Although this plant can be toxic when taken in very large doses, there is no danger as far as infusions are concerned.

Black hemp nettle alleviates palpitations and has a calming effect. Acting as a mild sedative, it helps soothe anxiety and nervousness related to psychological stress. Its only inconvenience is its bitter taste. For that reason, you should prepare a tincture instead of taking it in infusion form: Chop up a sufficient amount of fresh leaves and soak in an equal amount of 95-proof alcohol for two weeks. Filter and take 25 to 30 drops morning and night.

Common broom is often used as an ingredient in pharmaceutical preparations. Its active ingredient, sparteine, is extracted from leaves and stems and added to various drugs designed to regulate cardiac functions. Prepare infusions using only the buds—never more than a pinch per day, added to half a quart of boiling water, and infused for 15 minutes. If you develop any side effects (vomiting, dizziness, a slowing down of the pulse), stop taking the infusions immediately. These symptoms will only occur if you exceed the recommended dosage.

White horehound is a heart tonic that strengthens the cardiac muscle, helps combat fever, and stimulates appetite. Because its active ingredients are greatly weakened when the plant is dissolved in water, take capsules instead: three or four 0.5-gram capsules per day.

✎ Arteriosclerosis

Arteriosclerosis is a disease that makes the arteries begin to harden prematurely, usually because of unhealthy habits like tobacco or alcohol addiction, overeating, lack of exercise, and so on, and also by certain diseases like diabetes, hypertension, or obesity. Symptoms of arteriosclerosis include high blood pressure and insufficient circulation.

Lifestyle

Some basic changes in the way you live can make a big difference in the health of your arteries. Here are some great examples.

Get a move on. Exercise, as you know, is indispensable for maintaining good health. It becomes all the more important if you happen to be fighting

ARTERIOSCLEROSIS AND ATHEROSCLEROSIS ARE NOT THE SAME

Arteriosclerosis and atherosclerosis are often confused. While the two are similar, arteriosclerosis refers to a hardening of arteries that is generally characteristic of the aging process, while atherosclerosis refers to the formation of tumors filled with grainy matter.

Similar changes in lifestyle and nutrition are recommended for both conditions, but here are some plant remedies that especially target atherosclerosis.

• **Artichokes** are known to reduce levels of excess cholesterol and combat atherosclerosis. To prepare infusions, which you should drink before meals, add four or five grams of leaves to a liter of boiling water; filter and sweeten with honey to mask the bitter taste. You can also buy a commercially prepared tincture, which is less bitter tasting, in pharmacies: Take 50 to 100 drops a day.

• **Hawthorn** is a vasodilator and helps regulate cardiac functions. This plant is very beneficial for elderly persons suffering from a weak heart. It is also recommended for persons who are subject to a lot of professional stress. To prepare decoctions, soak two teaspoons of crushed flowers in a cup of cold water for seven or eight hours; bring to a boil and filter; drink one or two cups per day, in small sips. For infusions, use one teaspoon per cup of boiling water and let stand for 10 minutes; drink three or four cups a day.

• **Dandelion** helps cure circulatory disorders like hypertension, as well as liver and skin problems. It facilitates digestion and is recommended for diabetics. Soak 25 grams of chopped roots mixed with 25 grams of leaves in a liter of water for two hours; bring to a boil, then remove from heat and let stand for 20 minutes; drink a cup after meals. If you have an extractor, you can make your own dandelion juice, which is even more effective. Adding a tablespoon of fresh extract to a glass of milk makes an excellent tonic in spring, when fresh dandelions are readily available. Drink a glass or two every day.

a disease like arteriosclerosis. Ideally, exercise should be a part of your everyday routine, but it doesn't have to be an exhausting activity like long-distance running or jogging. Simply walking at a brisk pace or moderately strenuous bike riding will give you great results. You can also give your body a workout by leaving your car at home and walking to nearby destinations, or by climbing stairs instead of taking the elevator from time to time. If you don't exercise hard enough to work up a sweat, take a sauna or steam bath at least once a week.

Watch the pressure gauge. Keep a close eye on your blood pressure. Two quick ways to get your blood pressure down: Quit smoking, and try to organize your schedule to avoid any unnecessary stress.

Mind your attitude. The only real way to combat a disease like arteriosclerosis is to adopt a lifestyle that slows down the aging process. Of course that is easier said than done, but it is possible. Age is a question of attitude, as well as years: If you think of yourself as old, you will be more likely to act like an old person. Think young and you'll begin looking and feeling younger. That means always looking at life in terms of possibilities rather than limits.

Nutrition

As far as nutrition is concerned, try to cut down on the following foods: eggs, high-fat cheese, meat, and legumes that contain a lot of starch (beans, peas, lentils). Instead, eat more salads, low-fat cheeses, and natural rice and buckwheat, both of which help lower blood pressure and keep arteries and veins supple.

Also cut down on salt; use lemon instead of vinegar and herbs instead of hot spices. Steam your vegetables instead of boiling or frying them. Save those rich sauces for special occasions—in a relatively short time you'll feel so much better you won't crave them at all.

Gradually eliminate both tea and coffee, two stimulants you can do very well without. Try to avoid fat, especially animal fat, as much as possible. And use monounsaturated or polyunsaturated oil, like sesame seed, canola, and olive oils, when you cook, rather than saturated ones like lard and whole milk.

Butter is healthy as long as it is eaten raw, but don't use it to cook with too often and never allow it to turn black from overheating.

Plant Power

For keeping your arteries healthy, one plant food stands out among all the others:

Garlic is a delicious food, of course, but it also lowers blood pressure and keeps blood vessels supple, and has long been recognized as an effective prevention for hardening of the arteries. Add fresh raw garlic to salads and cooked foods, or prepare a garlic liqueur. Fill a glass container with fresh leaves or finely chopped bulbs (don't pack them in too tightly), then fill the container with 40-proof alcohol; let stand in direct sunlight or a warm location for at least two weeks. Take 10 to 15 drops in a little water, four times a day.

⬿ Arthritis

Unlike its more severe cousin rheumatoid arthritis (see Rheumatism), osteoarthritis is a disease that affects the cartilage in joints rather the bone itself or other organs. Healthy cartilage is a slippery substance that allows bones to slide over one another and acts as a kind of shock absorber between them. Osteoarthritis destroys that cartilage so that the bones underneath rub together, causing pain and swelling.

The causes of chronic osteoarthritis are varied and involve the entire body, rather than just one system or another. Factors like nutrition, hormonal imbalances, infection, intoxication, and lifestyle all play a role. For that reason, a holistic approach to healing is more likely to produce positive results than are localized treatments.

Because conventional medicine offers no cure, the disease has often been called a societal disorder, the result of negative habits linked to our modern lifestyle. And it is precisely by making certain changes to your lifestyle that you can hope to improve your condition.

General care

During crisis periods, here's a checklist of things you can do to relieve your pain and get back to normal:

- Wrap affected joints in a soft bandage and try to keep them as immobile as possible.
- From time to time, stimulate circulation in the affected joints by heating with a hair dryer or other device.
- Use the following three-day treatment: On the first day, wrap affected

joints in cabbage leaves that have been heated with an iron; on the second day, wrap joints in hot clay compresses; on the third day, apply a white cheese compress (see page 22 for instructions on making a compress).

- Take saunas on a regular basis if possible—heat has a beneficial effect on metabolism in general and can help combat disorders like osteoarthritis by eliminating accumulated toxins through the skin.

Nutrition

If there is one factor that is crucial for the prevention and treatment of osteoarthritis, it is proper nutrition. Some people have completely reversed the progress of the disease by changing their eating habits.

Get yourself used to eating natural, whole foods, such as whole grains, natural rice, fresh fruits and vegetables, and so on. At the same time eat fewer canned and processed foods and commercially prepared meals.

Unfortunately, if nothing tempts you more than a cheeseburger for lunch or a porterhouse steak for dinner, you may have to choose between the pleasures of your palate and your health, because research has established a definite link between premature aging and the amount of animal protein you ingest.

You can start by forgetting the idea that the more protein you eat, the healthier you will be. In the past, people were under the impression that they needed to ingest at least 100 to 200 grams of protein a day. This seems not to be the case. According to many experts, your daily protein requirement is in the area of 25 to 30 grams, not more.

So limit your protein intake, and try to get most of your daily requirement from vegetable proteins contained in foods like soy beans, sunflower seeds, almonds, millet, buckwheat, and nuts.

Here are a few other tips that will help you to conquer the pain of arthritis.

Drink your veggies. Replace your usual beverages with the water you use to cook potatoes, carrots or cabbage in. Potato juice is especially effective for the treatment of osteoarthritis.

Pollenate in the A.M. Every morning, eat a teaspoon of flower pollen along with your breakfast. This super-food is available in most health food stores. R. Chauvin, a nutrition expert and researcher, reports that pollen destroys harmful bacteria lodged in the intestines and facilitates digestion and elimination of waste.

Take Vitamin E. This vitamin has a beneficial effect on your general health, and will help regenerate damaged joints.

Plant Power

Here are some remedies from the plant world that can help to chase your arthritis pain away.

Burdock is especially effective if you happen to suffer from diabetes as well as osteoarthritis or rheumatism. Drink four or five cups of burdock infusion a day: Add 40 to 50 grams of fresh roots to a liter of boiling water and let stand for 10 minutes.

Chamomile can help soothe joint pain in some cases. Soak 30 grams of fresh or dried flowers in a liter of olive oil for 24 hours, then filter it and apply it locally as a massage oil.

Artichokes are diuretic and help eliminate bile. As such, they detoxify and can be effective in the fight against osteoarthritis. Prepare infusions by adding 4 or 5 grams of leaves to a liter of boiling water; sweeten with honey to neutralize the bitter taste, and drink a cup with your meals. If you find the taste of the infusion unpleasant, buy some tincture of artichoke at your local pharmacy or health food store; take 6 to 10 teaspoons a day, dissolved in water.

Marshmallow can be used as a mouthwash that helps combat osteoarthritis of the jaw. Add 50 grams of crushed leaves to a liter of cold water, bring to a boil, then let the brew stand for 10 minutes. Cool it to room temperature before using it.

Corn and millet can be used to prepare compresses that stay hot for a very long time (see how to prepare a compress on page 22). Applying hot compresses will stimulate circulation in affected joints, resulting in what is called hyperemia (greatly increased blood flow).

Mustard makes a poultice that is very effective for alleviating arthritic pain and increasing blood flow through affected joints.

Queen of the meadow is reputed to be a highly effective treatment for both osteoarthritis and rheumatism. In addition, the plant has a tonic effect on the heart. Drink between three and five cups of infusion a day: Pour a quarter of a liter of very hot (not boiling) water over the flower tops, and let it stand for a few minutes.

WHAT TO DO DURING AN ASTHMA ATTACK

If you happen to be around someone who is having a severe asthma attack, get the person to sit down, keeping his or her back straight and head up. Applying upward pressure on the lower stomach with both hands can help calm the person down. If no remedies are available, a cup of strong black cold coffee can help restore normal breathing.

Asthma

Asthma is a disorder that obstructs breathing passages, making breathing difficult. There are many possible causes and many types of asthma.

Any number of substances, from household dust to pet dander, can trigger allergy-related asthma.

Bronchial asthma, on the other hand, is often the result of changes in temperature. If a person whose respiratory system is already weakened by a pulmonary disorder develops asthma, the condition can be very difficult to cure.

Asthma attacks tend to be more frequent in the middle of the night. Persons wake up feeling as if they are suffocating. Attacks can last up to three hours and are often accompanied by violent coughing fits (children tend to wheeze instead of cough). The symptoms become more severe and more frequent as the disease develops.

General Care

During acute phases, asthma sufferers should stay in bed, in a well-ventilated, moderately heated room. If there are any pets in the house, they should be kept as far away from the sickroom as possible. Also try to eliminate as much dust as you can, by removing carpets, thick curtains, etc.

Most doctors prescribe some type of cortisone medication as a matter of course. Be very prudent when using them. New products are available that contain less cortisone, are just as effective, and are much less dangerous.

Children with asthma should not be overly protected or excluded from normal, day-to-day activities. Instead of improving their condition, over-protecting an asthmatic child can actually aggravate symptoms and make matters much worse later on. Children suffering from bronchial asthma should be given antispasmodic plant remedies.

Do your best to help asthma sufferers keep their spirits up. In some cases outside help, in the person of a psychotherapist or spiritual guide, might be worth a try. Autosuggestion can also be effective, especially in cases of chronic asthma.

Lifestyle

If you suffer from asthma, avoid exhausting sports that cause you to lose your breath. Smoking is extremely harmful: If you are asthmatic and a smoker, you should make every effort to quit. Here are some other helpful strategies.

Vacuum often. Your living space should be kept as clean and free of dust as possible. Always use a vacuum cleaner (professional quality, equipped with a HEPA filter if possible) instead of a broom to gather dust.

Get a new mattress. If you sleep on an old mattress, you should replace it. Persons suffering from cardiac-related asthma are advised to seek out a climate that is more conducive to preventing attacks, at least for the time it takes to get the condition under control (generally a period of two years without any attacks).

Charge the air. It's a good idea to keep a negative ion diffuser in your home. This device has proven effective in a large number of cases. Expect to wait three to six weeks before you start feeling the benefits. You can also inhale air directly as it flows out of the device: two 20-minute sessions per day.

Nutrition

Asthma sufferers should eat a regular, healthy diet consisting of light foods, low in protein and as natural as possible. Some suggestions include vegetable broth, fruit and vegetable stew, lots of fruit juice (orange, grape-fruit, lemon, tomato) accompanied by one or more of the herbal teas listed below. Make sure to get enough Vitamins A, B5, C, D, and E.

Avoid coffee and other stimulants.

Plant Power

Below are some powerful herbal remedies that can help you get your asthma under control.

Garlic is sometimes called natural penicillin; it is very useful for treating various types of pulmonary disorders. If you feel an attack coming on, put about 20 drops of garlic extract on a sugar cube and slowly suck on it.

To prepare your extract, simply soak a few average-size garlic cloves in some 90-proof alcohol for 10 days. Also make sure to use fresh garlic on a regular basis when preparing your meals.

Mullein helps alleviate coughing and has a sedative effect. It is especially recommended for elderly persons suffering from asthma. To prepare mullein infusions, add 1/3 oz of flowers to a quart of water and filter carefully with cotton or cheesecloth before drinking (fine hairs that are attached to the flowers can irritate your throat). Add honey to sweeten, and drink two or three cups per day.

Hyssop combats asthma, coughing, and other bronchial disorders. It is also a stimulant and an expectorant, helping eliminate bronchial secretions. Use 1/3 oz of flower tops per quart of boiling water, add honey to sweeten, and drink two or three cups a day.

Lavender acts as an antiseptic, antispasmodic, and sedative. Prepare infusions using 1 oz of flower tops per quart of boiling water, and inhale the rising steam during asthma attacks to open respiratory passages.

Ground ivy stimulates bronchial activity, so it's useful for all types of pulmonary disorders. The plant combats asthma, alleviates coughing, and helps cure emphysema. Drink three or four cups of ground ivy infusion per day, between meals: Use 1 oz of dried leaves per quart of boiling water, and let stand for 10 minutes.

Horehound alleviates coughing and works well for cases of asthma accompanied by lots of phlegm. Use 1 oz per quart of boiling water, let stand for 10 minutes, and drink three or four cups per day.

Butterburr is recommended for cases of bronchial asthma, and is amazingly effective for alleviating blocked breathing passages during attacks. Prepare an extraction by soaking a teaspoon of the plant in a cup of water overnight. You can also buy butterburr syrup in most pharmacies or health food stores.

Coltsfoot is an anti-inflammatory that has been successfully used for the treatment of bronchitis, bronchial asthma, and inflammation of the throat and trachea. If you are a smoker, you might want to try replacing tobacco with cigarettes made from coltsfoot. In addition to helping you break a harmful habit, inhaling the plant actually soothes the coughing fits that many smokers experience in the morning.

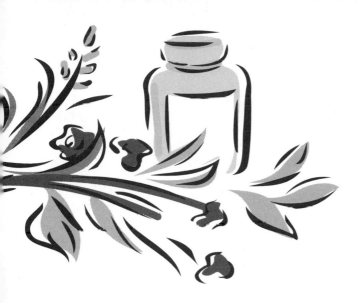

✍ Bleeding

The sight of blood pouring from a gash or a scrape can be frightening enough to send anyone into a panic. Yet sometimes even insignificant and superficial little cuts can produce copious bleeding. So how do you decide if a wound is serious enough to warrant a trip to the hospital?

Usually, bleeding from a wound is considered serious when it involves damage to a blood vessel. You can tell if that's happened by the flow and color of the blood. Here's all you need to know:

Injured artery: produces bright red blood and spurts with every heartbeat.

Injured vein: produces a flow of dark red.

Damaged capillary: oozes bright red blood from just under the surface of the skin.

Internal bleeding: can be detected by traces of blood in vomit, urine, or stool (either black or the color of port wine). Emergency medical care is a must.

Plant Power

Generally speaking you can rely on the plants mentioned below for the treatment of minor, external wounds and chronic internal bleeding that

HOW TO STOP A NOSEBLEED

Nosebleeds can be annoying, frightening, and difficult to stop. But with this simple three-step treatment, you should be able to halt the flow in no time.

- Take a teaspoon of shepherd's purse sap.
- Soak a strip of cotton in some fresh nettle juice and use it to plug the bleeding nostril. To obtain the juice, grind up some leaves and stems, boil them in a little water and then press them through some fine cotton or cheesecloth.
- Use cold horsetail decoctions in the same way once the bleeding has stopped.

you're managing under a doctor's supervision. For more serious problems, however, it's always best to consult a doctor. Some plants do have a powerful anti-bleeding effect, but these remedies should be prescribed by a specialist and used only under his or her supervision.

Yarrow can be helpful in stopping external bleeding. Apply ground leaves and flowers directly over the wound. If you cannot obtain fresh yarrow, use a decoction or ointment. Make a decoction by boiling 2 oz of dried leaves or flowers in a quart of water for 10 minutes. At the same time, drink infusions of horsetail and nettle to strengthen your organism: 2/3 oz of each per quart of water. To prepare yarrow ointment, use 2/3 oz each of finely chopped fresh yarrow and raspberry leaves, mixed with 3 oz of lard or petroleum jelly. Heat the mixture slightly, then let it stand overnight; next day heat it again slightly, filter it through some fine cheesecloth, and store it in a cold place. Apply this ointment directly to cuts.

Shepherd's purse is frequently prescribed for cases of internal hemorrhaging, because it acts on a substance called fibrine, a protein that helps speed up blood clotting. Use it to stop nosebleeds. Persons suffering from chronic internal bleeding (caused by an ulcer, for example) should take a teaspoon of shepherd's purse sap mixed with a cup of horsetail decoction each day for three months. A shepherd's purse and horsetail decoction can help cure bleeding from the kidneys: Boil 1 oz to 2 oz of dried plant in a quart of water for 10 minutes, and drink three small cups a day.

Nettle helps stop nosebleeds (see above), and is also recommended for cases of bronchial or uterine hemorrhaging, where blood is expelled through expectoration. Use 1 oz to 2 oz per quart of water to prepare infusions, and drink four cups a day.

Horsetail is very effective when combined with other anti-bleeding plants like yarrow or shepherd's purse. For external applications, prepare compresses using some freshly ground plant, or a concentrated decoction: Boil 3 oz in a quart of water for 15 minutes.

Marigold slows down blood flow when applied externally. Use the tincture (called Calendula by homeopathic specialists): Add one teaspoon to a cup of boiling water and let it cool. Or use a marigold ointment, applied directly to the cut.

✅ Blisters and Calluses

Have you ever gone for a long hike wearing a brand new pair of hiking boots or to a dance in a pair of stiff new dress shoes? If you have, you probably know what it feels like to suffer from painful blisters. Nothing will take you off your feet faster.

Plant Power

The best thing to do when blisters first start developing is to apply ice directly to the affected area. After that, it's time to turn to herbal remedies.

Chamomile can be made into a concentrated infusion (from 2 1/2 oz to 3 oz soaked in a quart of water for half an hour) and taken internally or used as a topical application.

Horsetail is excellent for soaking blistered feet or hands. Soak 2 oz of plant in a quart of cold water overnight; in the morning, bring to a boil (adding more water if necessary). Bathe affected areas for 20 minutes, then wrap them in cotton or gauze that has been soaked in the liquid for another 20 minutes.

Marigold is a good topical application for blisters that have opened: 1/2 oz per half quart of water, left to soak for half an hour.

Coltsfoot can provide significant relief. Apply fresh leaves directly to blisters.

❧ Breast-Feeding Problems

What could be more natural, nurturing, or expressive of the bond between a mother and her child than breast-feeding? Yet, as natural as it is, there are some do's and don'ts you should be aware of when you're providing your infant or toddler with the nourishment your own body produces.

Lifestyle

Remember, much of what you put into your own body travels in your breast milk to your infant's body. With that in mind, here are some things you should try to avoid.

Caffeine. As hard as it may be to do, this is a time in your life when you should avoid drinking coffee, tea, or soft drinks with caffeine in them. It can make your baby fussy.

Alcohol. Alcohol does pass through mother's milk, and can cause some serious problems in the developing nervous systems of newborns. It can also affect "letdown." So if you must drink, do so *moderately* and only *after* you've finished nursing, never before.

Tobacco. Nicotine does pass through breast milk, and can be a problem for your child if you smoke heavily. Any more than a pack a day can reduce your milk flow and harm your baby. If you must smoke, do so only after you've nursed, and be sure to stay well away from your infant or toddler while you're doing it. Second-hand smoke is even more harmful to babies than to other adults.

Medications. Try to avoid any medicine that contains an antihistamine, unless it's marked "non-drowsy formula." Antihistamines can reduce your milk supply. Check with your doctor before taking any other medications.

Gas producers. Foods like onions, cabbage, broccoli, and beans may make your baby fussy.

Plant Power

There are a number of plants that stimulate milk production in mothers of newborn infants. The following list, although not exhaustive, offers a variety of botanicals from which you can choose.

Angelica is a mild stimulant that serves as a general tonic and fortifier.

It also helps regulate stomach functions. Prepare decoctions by boiling 1 oz of roots in a quart of water for five minutes (or a 1/2 oz mixture of leaves and seeds for two minutes).

Green aniseed helps alleviate stomach problems and excess gas. Drink two or three cups of infusion per day, before or after meals: 1/2 oz of seeds per quart of water.

Caraway is a stimulant and diuretic. It also regulates the secretion of bile from the gall bladder. Drink a cup of infusion after meals: 1/3 oz of seeds per quart of water; infuse for 10 minutes.

Cumin facilitates digestion. Prepare infusions using 1/3 oz of seeds per quart of water; let stand for 10 minutes and drink a cup after meals.

Fennel is a diuretic that stimulates menstrual flow and aids digestion. Drink three or four cups of decoction per day: Boil 1 oz of roots or seeds in a quart of water (roots for five minutes, seeds for three minutes); remove from heat and let stand for 10 minutes.

Fenugreek is a fortifier that also stimulates lactation. Prepare decoctions by boiling 1 oz to 2 oz of seeds in a quart of water for 10 minutes. You can also buy fenugreek extract at most pharmacies and health food stores. Some people prefer it because of the plant's unusual taste.

Hops stimulate appetite, facilitate digestion, and act as a mild sedative and depurative. Use 1/2 oz of cones per quart of water to prepare infusions.

Pimpernel can be ground up and applied as a poultice on the breasts. It's reputed to stimulate lactation.

BREAST ENGORGEMENT

This problem generally affects pregnant or breast-feeding mothers, although a breast ulcer is a possible cause. If the problem is an ulcer (engorgement will be accompanied by oscillating fever and more intense pain), see a doctor as soon as possible. If it's common engorgement, however, try these tips to get relief.

Soothe with mint. Mint helps alleviate painful, engorged breasts; simply apply fresh mint leaves as poultices.

Apply parsley. Parsley also helps alleviate engorgement: Use fresh leaves as poultices.

Try horsetail. Heat up some horsetail in a double boiler and apply as hot compresses to alleviate engorged breasts.

BREAST CARE

Firm, healthy, and youthful: Those are the three watchwords of breast care. And likewise there are three plants that can help you give your breasts the care they need.

Yarrow helps keep breasts youthful. Using an infusion can help eliminate wrinkles on the breasts. Infuse 1/2 oz of plant in a quart of water. Drink two or three cups a day, and apply compresses soaked in freshly extracted juice. If you cannot obtain the fresh plant, boil 2 oz of yarrow in a quart of water for 10 minutes, cool and apply as compresses.

Fennel keeps breasts firm. If you want to prevent sagging, infuse 1/2 oz of powdered seeds in one cup of boiled water for a few minutes; cool and apply. This plant also helps reduce swelling of engorged breasts: Cook a handful of plant, then grind it up and apply locally.

Goat's rue keeps breasts healthy. It's reputed to stimulate milk production in nursing mothers. Boil 1/2 oz of plant in half a quart of water for 10 minutes; mix with clay, and apply directly to the breasts. You can also drink a cup of goat's rue infusion (available in teabags) morning and night.

➣ Bronchitis

You can always spot people with bronchitis—they sound as if they're about to cough themselves inside out. At the very least, they tend to wheeze or whistle when they breathe and can produce considerable phlegm as the mucous membranes in their breathing passages become inflamed.

Bronchitis can be either chronic or acute. The acute variety, which tends to affect children and elderly persons, is accompanied by slight fever, aches and pains, and sometimes by a feeling of mild depression. Coughing up phlegm is common, and pain sometimes occurs in the muscles in the center of the chest. Coughing generally lasts for one or two weeks. In case of high fever or extreme difficulty breathing, consult a doctor as soon as possible.

Chronic bronchitis produces the same symptoms as the acute type, but recurs once or twice a year. Smokers are especially susceptible to this form of the disease.

A doctor may prescribe antibiotics, but that doesn't mean you can't take steps on your own to cure the problem.

General Care

During acute attacks, bronchitis sufferers should stay in bed, especially if they have a high fever. Maintain an ambient temperature of 65 degrees Fahrenheit in the sickroom, and make sure air circulation is adequate. Use mustard baths for the feet and spray the sickroom with eucalyptus.

Bronchitis sufferers should, of course, avoid smoking.

Nutrition

The ideal diet for bronchitis sufferers should be natural, light, and easy to digest. Avoid foods rich in refined carbohydrates (white sugar, white flour, etc.), cut down on dairy products, and steer clear of alcohol and coffee.

Plant Power

If hacking, coughing, and wheezing are making your life a misery, try some of these herbal recipes. You may be pleasantly surprised.

Angelica is recommended for all types of respiratory ailments, especially those that affect children. It's an effective stimulant and fortifier. Prepare infusions using 1/2 oz of roots or seeds per quart of boiling water, and infuse for 10 minutes. Drink four cups a day.

Mullein is an expectorant, so it helps you bring up phlegm and open breathing passages. It also has a calming effect and promotes sleep. Prepare infusions using 1/2 oz of flowers per quart of boiling water, and let stand for 10 minutes. Filter, add a little honey to taste, and drink two cups per day.

Borage helps combat fever and alleviates inflammation of the respiratory passages. Prepare infusions using 2 or 3 teaspoons of dried leaves per cup of boiling water; let stand for five minutes, filter, and sweeten with honey. Drink two cups a day for a week.

Eucalyptus is often used as an inhalant to help stop coughing and open breathing passages. Boil 1 oz of shredded eucalyptus leaves in a quart of water for 10 minutes. Pour the liquid into an inhaler (a device that you can buy at most pharmacies or health food stores), or lean over the pot with a towel over your head and breathe in the steam. Repeat three times a day. To disinfect the sickroom, use a portable stove to boil a mixture of eucalyptus leaves, black poplar buds, and pine cones; add a teaspoon of turpentine, drop by drop, until all the water has evaporated. You can also use a eucalyptus decoction to combat coughing: Boil 2/3 oz of leaves in a quart of water for one minute; let it stand for 10 minutes, filter, and add a little honey. Drink five cups a day.

Marshmallow helps stops coughing and decongests your air passageways. Soak a teaspoon of leaves, stems, or roots in a cup of cold water for eight hours; filter and heat slightly before drinking; have one cup per day.

Ground ivy is prescribed for all types of disorders of the lungs and breathing passages, especially chronic bronchitis. Use decoctions: Boil 1 oz of flowers in a quart of water for about 15 minutes; filter, sweeten with a little honey, and drink four cups a day.

Horehound is useful in fighting both chronic and acute bronchitis. The plant helps stop coughing and aids the body in getting rid of phlegm. Use infusions: Add about 1 oz to a quart of boiling water; let stand for 10 minutes, and sweeten with honey. Drink at least five cups a day.

Mustard poultices have long been used to alleviate chest congestion. Prepare a paste with 12 oz of finely ground mustard seeds mixed with an equal amount of linseed flour; add some lukewarm water, and apply the paste directly on the chest. Foot baths also help decongest airways. Use one cup of mustard seeds per quart of very hot water, and soak the feet for 10 or 15 minutes.

Horsetail is a tonic for the lungs and is often recommended for cases of chronic bronchitis. To prepare infusions, add 2 teaspoons of dried plant to 1/2 cup of boiling water and let it stand for a few minutes. Drink one cup a day.

Coltsfoot has long been used to treat bronchitis. It quiets coughing and helps you clear out phlegm. Persons suffering from chronic bronchitis or dry cough can smoke coltsfoot cigarettes, made with leaves that are slightly fermented. Coltsfoot cigarettes contain no tar or nicotine, so smokers can use them to replace ordinary cigarettes and give their lungs a break. You can also prepare coltsfoot infusions: Use about 1 oz of leaves per quart of boiling water. Let the brew stand for half an hour, filter, and add honey to taste. Drink four cups a day.

≫ Bruises

They're ugly, they hurt, and some of us seem more prone to them than others. Bruises, or contusions, come from blows, strong pressure, or prolonged friction delivered to the skin. In fact, the characteristic purple color is caused by small blood vessels bursting beneath the surface of the skin. The only real difference between a cut and a bruise is that the skin covering a bruise does not open.

Contusions can be treated effectively at home. There's no need to consult a doctor unless you suspect that a bone has been fractured or that internal bleeding of some kind is taking place.

Plant Power

Apply cold compresses to the affected area, followed by compresses made with one or another of the plants listed below.

Arnica is an extremely effective treatment for bruises of all kinds, producing astonishing results in some cases. It's especially recommended for muscles that remain stiff and sore for days after bruising occurs. Always keep a 4-oz bottle of Arnica tincture handy for external applications. To prepare compresses, simply soak a piece of gauze or cotton with tincture and apply it to the affected area. *Important: Do not use arnica on open wounds.* To prepare infusions, add 1/2 oz of arnica to 6 oz of boiling water; remove from heat and let stand for 10 minutes. Soak a piece of sterilized cotton in the preparation, smear a little lard or petroleum jelly on the material, and place over the bruise (cover with plastic if clothes are to be worn over the compress).

Rose and thyme are applied externally: Fill a linen bag with rose or thyme, heat in the oven, and apply to the bruise.

Marigold makes an excellent ointment for treating bruises. Put 1 oz of flowers or dried leaves through a blender (you can also use one teaspoon of freshly extracted juice); simmer 1 oz of lard or petroleum jelly until liquid and stir in the marigold. Remove it from the heat, and filter it through a piece of linen or cotton, then let it stand for a day. Store the ointment in clean glass or ceramic pots.

∾ Burns

Burns are among the injuries we fear most, and with good reason. They're terribly painful, they become easily infected, and, in extreme cases, they can be lethal. Whether a burn is minor or major, speed is of the utmost importance in treating it.

For localized minor burns, apply cold compresses or soak affected areas in cold water, if no other remedies are available. But *don't* use ice. It can damage the skin.

For more serious or widespread burns, wrap the person in a clean sheet and take him or her to the nearest hospital as quickly as possible. Burns are considered serious when the skin is open (second-degree burn). For acid burns, disinfect the wound thoroughly *before* treating.

Plant Power

The medicinal power of plants can seem almost miraculous when applied

---

A BURN ISN'T JUST A BURN

The way a burn is treated depends on how deeply it has damaged the skin. Here's how you can judge, at a glance, just how serious a burn injury is.

- **First-degree burns,** such as sunburn, are moist, red, and painful. As a rule, they don't blister, and they usually heal within a week.
- **Second-degree burns** sear off the top layer of skin and penetrate to the under-layer (the dermis). They can be either superficial or deep. Superficial burns affect only the top of the dermis. They are extremely painful, especially when touched, and moist. The skin may develop a patchy pink or red appearance, and often blisters. Superficial second-degree burns usually heal on their own. Deep second-degree burns penetrate farther into the dermis. They're usually painful, and they often look pale and dry. They can take up to a month to heal, and they often leave significant scarring.
- **Third-degree burns** go all the way through the skin. The burned area is blackened and leathery. Oddly, these burns are often not painful because the nerve endings that cause pain have been seared off. Healing doesn't take place without skin grafts.

to the sting of a burn. Not only do they promote rapid healing, but they also soothe away pain. Here are some to have on hand in case of emergency.

Aloe vera rapidly alleviates pain caused by minor burns and is an effective treatment against infection. If you have an aloe plant growing in your home, cut a piece of bottom leaf, peel off the skin, and place it directly on the burn. When the pulp dries, scratch the leaf with a knife and more sap will appear.

Mullein decoctions can be used to make dressings: Soak three handfuls of flowers and leaves in a quart of cold water overnight; then soak gauze in the liquid and dress the wound.

Carrots can also be used to soothe pain caused by burns: Simply grate a carrot and apply directly to the affected area.

> ## CARING FOR A SUNBURN
>
> **A** nasty sunburn can ruin your whole vacation, not to mention that it ages your skin and puts you at greater risk for skin cancer. It's best to avoid overexposure to the sun in the first place, either by covering up or by using a sunscreen with an SPF of 15 or higher, but even if you're already burned there's something you can do: Try one of these remedies.
>
> **Linden** baths have an immediately soothing effect and tone the skin. Pour two quarts of infusion (2 oz of plant per two quarts of water) into the bath before adding your bath water.
>
> **Aloe vera** is an extremely effective treatment for all kinds of burns, including sunburns. Apply pure gel (available in some pharmacies and most health food stores) to affected areas.

St. John's wort is used to prepare an oil that is effective for treating burns. The oil should be prepared in advance, and stored away for emergencies. Fill a glass container with St. John's wort, then cover with extra virgin olive oil. Seal the container and let it stand in direct sunlight, or near a heat source, for five or six weeks, agitating the mixture from time to time. When the oil takes on a distinct red color, filter and store in an opaque container (the oil can be kept for up to two years). Use as an external application for open cuts and wounds, bruises, and burns.

Potatoes are more than just delicious—they can also be therapeutic! To treat minor burns, peel and slice a raw potato and apply it directly to the affected area for rapid relief. *Do not use this remedy on burns where the skin has opened or on acid burns, as bacteria from the potato can cause an infection.*

Marigold in a tincture or decoction makes an excellent treatment for both burns and cuts. To prepare a decoction, boil a pinch in a quart of water for 10 minutes. To prepare a tincture, soak a cup of flowers in a quart of 40-proof alcohol for a few days, placing the container in direct sunlight or near some other heat source.

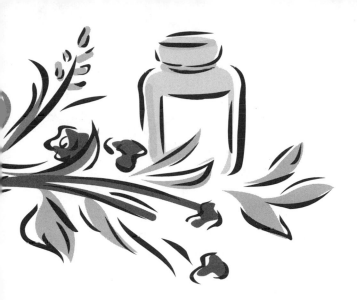

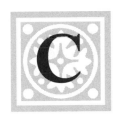

☙ Cancer

We're all looking for miracles, but even after decades of research, cancer remains a major killer that resists our best efforts to find a cure. So whenever the 6 o'clock news breaks a story that some common herb has been magically healing people at clinics in the Bahamas or Mexico, it's hard not to get excited—at least until the skeptics begin debunking and the experts begin debating. Then we don't know what to believe.

Is it even possible? Can herbal remedies really achieve what the best minds in medical research have been trying to do for decades? Well, the answer is yes…and no. We're not suggesting that any of the remedies included in this section will work miracles. But it does seem true that plants have, in some cases, cured cancer after all attempts at conventional medical treatment have failed.

How? We don't know. While specialists agree that diet, lack of physical activity, mood, heredity, viruses, repeated local inflammation, and over 600 known carcinogens can each play a role in causing the disease, no one really understands cancer well enough to say how the occasional surprise cure happens.

We do know enough, however, to make some suggestions about preventing the disease and about how to help tip the odds in your favor if you already have it.

Lifestyle

Most health experts agree that emotions have a profound affect on health. Some go even further, claiming that developing a sense of joie de vivre is crucial for maintaining a strong, effective immune system.

Here are some ways in which you can change your lifestyle that will help you prevent—or even recover—from this devastating disease.

Be positive. Time and time again, attitude has proven an important factor in the healing process. Patients with a positive outlook recover more rapidly than those who are depressed or ridden with anxiety.

Relax a little. Take time out for yourself and do something you enjoy, like gardening or baking. Autosuggestion and meditation also help bring out the best in us, and help us maintain a positive state of mind.

Perk up your living quarters. Living in a bright, well-ventilated house or apartment has been shown to stimulate people's lymphatic and immune systems.

Work out for health. Exercise whenever the opportunity arises, and try your best to stop smoking if you happen to be addicted to cigarettes.

Turn up the heat. Saunas are very beneficial for persons suffering from cancer and arthritis, as a large number of toxins are eliminated through perspiration. Try to take at least two sauna baths per week.

Nutrition

An improper diet is one of the factors known to be responsible for a number of types of cancer. Here are some dietary changes that can help you prevent this disease.

Avoid yellow food coloring. Used to make margarine look like butter, this common dye causes cancer in rats, unless their diet also contains wheat, powdered liver, or brewer's yeast.

Avoid animal protein. Consuming too much has been linked to an increased incidence of cancer. The United States, where people consume more animal protein than in any other country, has the highest incidence of cancer, as well as arthritis, diabetes, and heart disease.

Go easy on the salt. The World Health Organization reported that the incidence of stomach cancer in Japan was linked to an excessive intake of refined salt.

Go organic. Shop for organic fruit and vegetables, grown without chemical fertilizers or pesticides, whenever possible, and make sure to wash your fruits and vegetables thoroughly. Some of these chemicals are suspected of being human carcinogens.

Cut out acids. If you suffer from leukemia, avoid acidic fruits and vegetables like lemons, oranges, V-8 juice, and so on, as well as spicy, salty foods, fat meat, and/or processed meats.

Plant Power

Below are some plants that may help you in the battle against cancer. But remember, we are in no way suggesting that taking herbs is meant to replace the care of a qualified physician, and we do not wish to encourage anyone to develop false hope. Unless medical researchers come up with some breakthrough discovery, cancer

SO WHAT CAN I EAT?

Fortunately, in contrast to the growing list of foods that are suspected of causing cancer, a number of foods actually help prevent the disease.

Research in the United States has shown that garlic can be effective for preventing the formation of cancer tumors. Taking large doses of Vitamin C on a regular basis also helps fight the spread of free radicals, cells that are responsible for the formation of tumors.

Other foods that can help fight cancer include red beets, raw carrots, raw spinach, fresh fruits, parsley, and tarragon. When using oil, always opt for first cold-pressed corn, sesame, or sunflower seed oil, and use honey instead of sugar as a sweetener whenever possible. Sesame butter, which contains up to 43 percent unsaturated fatty acids, facilitates digestion.

Brewer's yeast, wheat germ, and magnesium, found in unrefined sea salt, are all recommended. Sprinkle a teaspoon of brewer's yeast on salads, soups, and desserts as often as you can, and add wheat germ to your morning cereal or fruit juice every day.

is and will remain a disease that is very difficult to cure. We simply encourage you to take responsibility for your own health and to explore any avenue that offers the possibility of improving your chances for survival. Plants do not offer an alternative to chemotherapy or radiation therapy, but they may be a valuable adjunct to your treatment.

One final caution: Always let your doctor know if you're using any of these remedies. He or she can help you avoid having any unwanted drug/herb interactions.

Yarrow can be combined with horsetail to combat lung cancer: Mix four cups of yarrow infusion with one cup of horsetail infusion (see below), and add another half cup later on in the day. Also chew sweet flag root, and wash down the juice with a cup of yarrow tea. Preparation: Half an ounce of plant per half quart of boiling water.

Celandine stimulates liver functions and can help combat cancer because this organ is often affected by the disease.

Bedstraw has been used with some success to treat cancer of the tongue. Prepare infusions by adding one teaspoon of bedstraw to two cups of boiling water. Fresh bedstraw sap, mixed with butter, helps combat mouth ulcers and lesions. Make sure to have any unusual lesion checked by a doctor before trying to treat it yourself.

Mistletoe has a beneficial effect on the body's overall metabolism; is commonly used to treat hypertension, arthritis, and arteriosclerosis; and can help prevent or combat cancer. Mistletoe tincture is available in pharmacies and health food stores.

Lapacho is used by South American healers to prevent and cure all types of cancer, including leukemia. Add the entire contents of one or two droppers to a cup of water and drink. Take three times a day. As a preventive measure, take 20 drops a day.

Lycopodium (club moss) is used to treat cancer of the liver, a difficult type of cancer to treat under any circumstances. Drink a cup of infusion in the morning before breakfast and another a half hour before your evening meal. Complete with depurative and horsetail compresses (see entries).

Marjoram is recommended for combating cancer of the lymph glands. Fill a glass container with fresh marjoram (don't pack too tightly) and cover with extra virgin olive oil. Soak in direct sunlight or near a heat source for 10 days. Apply the oil to affected glands, alternating with marigold ointment (see below) and St. John's wort oil.

Nettle is often prescribed as a depurative, and can help cure cancer of the spleen when taken as a cure over a period of some weeks. Make sure not to boil nettle infusions: Add a teaspoon to a cup of previously boiled water, and let stand for three minutes. Nettle can also be combined with an equal amount of marigold to combat stomach cancer. Sip the mixture throughout the course of the day, and complete the treatment with depurative compresses. Nettle infusions are also helpful for healing surgical wounds: Apply locally, along with horsetail compresses that have been heated with steam.

Butterburr cannot cure cancer, but it does have anticarcinogenic properties and helps alleviate cramps and pain. You can ingest large amounts of this completely nontoxic plant on a daily basis, along with your meals. For cancer of the lymph glands, prepare poultices: Take some freshly washed butterburr, St. John's wort, bedstraw and marigold leaves; crush them, while still wet, with a rolling pin. Cover affected glands with the resulting paste. If you have to undergo surgery, use the depurative infusion described earlier to prepare compresses, to accelerate healing.

Horsetail is reputed to stop the growth of tumors, and in some cases causes them to shrink. It can also be used to prepare steam-heated compresses to alleviate pain and accelerate healing after surgery. Heat your horsetail leaves in a double boiler; once the leaves have softened, wrap them in a thick woolen cloth and apply firmly to affected areas so that they retain their heat; leave in place for at least two hours. Horsetail also helps prevent cancer, especially lung cancer, when combined with yarrow. To prepare a decoction, boil 2 oz of dried stems in a quart of water for 10 minutes.

Sweet flag is recommended for the treatment of intestinal cancer and leukemia. Place a teaspoon of roots in a cup of cold water and soak overnight; filter, heat, and drink six mouthfuls a day (no more) before and after meals. You can also combine sweet flag and marigold.

Marigold is known to prevent cancer of the stomach and uterus. Use macerations: Soak 30 grams of leaves and flowers in a quart of cold water overnight; drink two cups per day. Maria Treben, a renowned herbal therapist, recommends the following remedy for combating tumors in the lower stomach, ovaries and uterus: six to eight teaspoons of depurative tea (see Appendix A) diluted in 1.5 quarts of herbal tea made from 10 oz of marigold and an equal amount of yarrow. She also recommends taking yarrow sitz baths three times a week. For cancer of the intestines or pancreas, as well as for leukemia, mix 6 oz of marigold, 3 1/2 oz of yarrow and 3 1/2 oz of nettle; add 6 teaspoons of the mixture to 1.5 quarts of water and bring to a boil; drink a mouthful every 15 minutes to facilitate digestion. You can also add a tablespoon of depurative tea to half a cup of the mixture; drink half before your main meal of the day, and the other half after the meal. Or soak some soft material in the depurative tea remedy and apply to the stomach area. Marigold ointment is helpful for combating cancer of the lymph glands: Put two heaping cups of leaves, stems, and flowers through a blender; add to 1 lb of melted lard (keep the cooking temperature under 100 degrees centigrade); remove from heat, filter through cheesecloth or linen, and let stand for a day; filter again through a fine cotton cloth and store in opaque glass or plastic containers; apply as needed to affected areas.

≈ Cataracts

This is a common disorder of the eyes, and, if left untreated, a dangerous one. The symptoms are obvious: The lens of the eye gradually grows more and more opaque, resulting in foggy or fuzzy vision and, eventually, blindness. Conventional medical treatments consist of eye lotions to slow down the growth of cataracts and surgery when vision becomes severely limited.

Plant Power

Fortunately, this is one area in which you can do some real good with medicinal plants, such as the one mentioned below. They can inhibit the growth of cataracts and postpone the need for surgery.

Celandine is sometimes effective in impeding the growth of cataracts. Put some fresh leaves through a juicer or blender and dab the juice on your closed eyelids. If you cannot obtain fresh juice, use a few drops of commercially prepared celandine tincture instead. A depurative infusion can help if the disorder is at an early stage of development. Put a few drops in the corners of the eyes, or apply compresses soaked in the mixture. Repeat daily.

Note: Two homeopathic remedies, Calcium fluoratum and Kalium chloratum, are also effective for the treatment of cataracts. Consult a specialist for more details.

🌿 Cellulite

Cellulite, that puckery fat that mottles the skin of the hips, thighs, and butt, isn't really dangerous, of course, but that doesn't mean it's lovable either. Most women (the problem affects women almost exclusively) would love to get rid of their cellulite if they could.

There are a number of solutions available, ranging from specialized diets and exercise programs to costly spa treatments and surgical interventions like liposuction. Unfortunately, there is no guarantee that any of these interventions will work. Regular exercise and a balanced diet are still the best ways to reduce or eliminate localized areas of cellulite.

THE SEVEN WARNING SIGNS OF CATARACTS

According to the U.S. Department of Health and Human Services, your eyes give you plenty of warning when cataracts are developing. Here are the symptoms to be aware of:

- Cloudy, fuzzy, foggy, or filmy vision
- Changes in the way you see colors
- Problems driving at night because headlights seem too bright
- Problems with glare from lamps or the sun
- Frequent changes in your eyeglass prescription
- Double vision
- Better near vision for a while (only in farsighted people)

Lifestyle

There are exercises you can do that help get rid of cellulite (flutter kicking in a swimming pool, climbing a stairmaster, stationary bicycling, or any other exercise that challenges the leg muscles and burns fat). Spas offer algae baths and massages with special devices made of wooden balls. Using a rough washing glove in the shower is helpful, as are certain skin creams.

Nutrition

Changing your diet won't completely eliminate cellulite, but it can help. Here are some places to start.

Make your diet hypotoxic. That means cut down on tea, coffee, alcohol, pastry, processed meats, sugar, and very sweet fruits. Recommended fruits include melon, pineapple, strawberries, and grapefruit.

Fast occasionally. Go on a one-day fast every three months to allow your body to eliminate toxins and some excess fat.

Hydrate. Drink one or two quarts of spring water (with a low mineral content) every day between meals. Eat a lot of grated carrots, cooked artichokes (seasoned with a little oil and lemon), fresh lettuce, and lemons (raw or cooked).

Plant Power

Below are some plants you can use to speed along the effects of your diet and exercise program by helping to eliminate excess fluids, which can worsen the appearance of cellulite. But don't expect magic. You may see improvement, but carrying a little cellulite is so common that it should be considered normal.

Birch has a diuretic effect and helps stimulate digestion. Prepare infusions using 1/2 oz of leaves per quart of boiling water and let stand for 15 minutes. Filter and add the juice of two lemons and a little bicarbonate of soda. Drink the mixture throughout the day and with meals.

Broom heather improves blood circulation and acts as a diuretic. You can combine it with queen of the meadow and couchgrass (also called dog-grass): Mix one ounce of broom heather with 1/2 oz of queen of the meadow and couchgrass, and boil in a quart of water for one minute. Drink the preparation throughout the day, between meals.

Climbing ivy and celandine can be combined in an external application that softens thickened skin and helps dissolve fat. Put 50 grams of each plant in a quart of water and boil for three minutes. Soak compresses in the liquid and apply while they are still hot.

Kelp stimulates endocrine functions and regularizes the metabolism of fats. Massage affected areas with fresh kelp, ideally imported directly from the seaside. You can also drink three or four cups of kelp decoction per day, before meals, to help eliminate cellulite on the hips, nape of the neck, and midriff: Boil 1/2 oz of kelp in a quart of water for five minutes; expect to wait two or three weeks before seeing any results.

≋ Colds

According to some estimates, one billion cold infections occur in the United States every year. So pretty much everyone is familiar with the symptoms: scratchy throat, sneezing, maybe a slight fever, headaches, coughing, and the inevitable nasal drip.

Colds rarely last longer than 8 to 10 days. Although generally benign, these infections should be treated in order to avoid the risk of serious complications like sinus or middle ear infections.

General Care

In most cases it isn't necessary to see a doctor if you think you have a common cold. Many of the plant remedies listed below are surprisingly effective for alleviating symptoms and accelerating healing. Don't use nasal drops to excess, because they can have a "rebound" effect, which will actually worsen your symptoms.

Chamomile vapor can help alleviate cold symptoms. Add 1 oz of leaves and flowers to a quart of boiling water; lean over the pot, head covered with a towel or a large piece of material, and inhale the steam for as long as you can. To clear nasal passages, mix 2 oz of chamomile with 2 oz of thyme; add a pinch of the mixture to 1/2 cup of boiling water, cool and use to rinse the nasal passages.

Borage soothes inflammation of the breathing passages and stimulates perspiration. Infuse 1 oz of dried plant in a quart of boiled water for five minutes, and drink four or five cups a day.

Eucalyptus reduces fever and has an antiseptic effect. Use 1 oz of leaves per quart of water to prepare infusions, and let stand for 15 minutes; add a little lemon juice to taste and drink four to six cups a day.

Eyebright can be used to prepare a tincture that irrigates nasal passages. Soak 1 oz of crushed plant in 1 cup of 70-proof alcohol for eight days. Use 25 to 30 drops per nostril to clear nasal passages.

Ground ivy alleviates coughing and soothes irritated mucous membranes in the nose and throat. Prepare infusions using 1 oz of flower tops per quart of water, add a pinch of aniseed to neutralize the bitter taste, and drink four or five cups a day (or use as a gargle). To clear blocked nasal passages, use infusions or freshly pressed juice.

Malva soothes inflammation and alleviates coughing. Infuse 1 oz of dried leaves or flowers in a quart of water for 20 minutes, and drink four to six cups a day. You can also combine 2 pinches of malva and 1 oz of pine buds; add a few cloves to taste, and use a tablespoon of the mixture per cup of boiling water to prepare infusions; drink two or three cups a day.

Onion is a popular remedy for common colds. Simply cut a slice of onion, soak it in a cup of hot water for a couple of minutes, then sip the liquid. Onion compresses also help clear stuffy nasal passages: Hold a slice up to your nose, or leave a couple of slices on your night table while you sleep.

Fir balsam is a diuretic and antiseptic that is recommended for all bronchial disorders including persistent colds. Add 1 oz of buds to a quart of boiling water, and let stand for half an hour; drink two or three cups a day.

Thyme can be mixed with eucalyptus and rosemary to make a very effective remedy for unblocking nasal passages. Use 2 oz of thyme and rosemary and 1 oz of eucalyptus; put about an ounce of the mixture into a quart of boiling water and inhale the steaming vapor (drape a towel or large piece of material over your head and the water to create a collecting "tent" for the vapors).

Coltsfoot alleviates coughing and facilitates expectoration. Use 2 oz of flowers per quart of water to prepare infusions, and drink three cups a day.

∼ Colic (Also See Hepatic Colic, Renal Colic)

Colic is infamous for making babies wail and giving parents sleepless nights. But it can happen to adults, as well.

It's that sharp, crampy feeling you sometimes get in your lower abdomen, caused by spasms of the colon, which in turn obstruct digestion. When you have that feeling, the first thing you should do is consult a doctor in order to make sure that the problem really is colic, and not a more serious disorder like hernia or appendicitis. But if colic is the diagnosis, there's lots you can do.

Plant Power

Here are some remedies from herbal lore that take that wretched feeling out of your tummy and put a smile back on your face.

Absinthe stimulates digestive functions and corrects digestive problems. To prepare infusions, use a pinch per cup of boiling water. Aniseed is a general stimulant which also helps alleviate problems caused by intestinal gas, a swollen belly, or constipation. It also has an analgesic, soothing effect. Prepare infusions using one teaspoon of seeds per cup of boiling water. *Note: Breast-feeding mothers should not use this remedy.*

Chamomile helps alleviate colic caused by intestinal gas, facilitates digestion, and soothes stomach cramps. Use chamomile extract as a stomach rub, or drink infusions: 1/2 oz of flowers per quart, infused for one-half hour.

Marshmallow alleviates irritation and inflammation. It's an effective treatment for colic, as well as diarrhea and constipation. To prepare infusions, add 1 oz of flowers to a quart of boiling water. For cases of chronic colic, soak 1 oz of roots in a quart of water overnight, at room temperature; sweeten with honey to neutralize the bitter taste.

Malva lessens cramping and combats constipation. Use a decoction: Boil 2/3 oz of flowers in a quart of water for 10 or 15 minutes.

✎ Colitis

Symptoms of a colon infection include diarrhea, intestinal colic, sometimes a fever, and persistent pain, either on the right or left side of the abdominal area.

Consult a doctor, naturopath, or homeopath to confirm the diagnosis. In addition to infections of bacterial origin, the condition can also be triggered by the use of antibiotics, in which case stool may have a firmer consistency, resembling paste, and take on an orange color.

Nutrition

A proper diet is extremely important when fighting colitis. The wrong foods, on the other hand, can make the condition worse. Here are some suggestions for making your meals work to make you feel better.

Start with liquids. During acute attacks, limit your food intake to unsalted vegetable broth. As you begin feeling better, add some quince or bilberry jam on toast, carrot soup, cooked rice with a little sugar, and carob and flour pudding.

Eat more than an apple a day. Going on an apple cure for a few days (1 lb of grated apples, with peel, per day) can be very beneficial.

Easy on the starch. If stool is pale and acidic, with the consistency of paste, eliminate flour and other starchy foods, fermented cheese, and raw vegetables like cabbage, radishes and cucumbers. Stop eating spicy foods for a couple of weeks as well.

Boycott animal products. If stool has a very dark color, eliminate meat, milk, and other dairy products. Once you're feeling better, if you feel you must eat meat, grill it and be sure it's a lean cut.

Plant Power

Here are some herbal remedies that can ease the misery of colitis.

Aloe vera has a toning and regularizing effect on the entire digestive system. Drink one or two tablespoons of pure aloe vera juice or gel (available in health food stores) a day. If you happen to have an aloe plant growing around the house, cut off one of the fleshy lower leaves, place the peel in a little water, and store in your fridge; drink a couple of mouthfuls twice a week.

Cabbage alleviates irritation and helps heal lesions in the stomach and intestines. Drink two glasses of fresh cabbage juice per day, between meals, for three weeks out of every month.

Savory makes an effective remedy for diarrhea and difficult digestion. It also acts as an antiseptic to combat infection. Prepare infusions using 2 oz per quart of water, and drink as needed.

Thyme is an antiseptic that promotes better elimination of toxins. It also has a tonic and antispasmodic effect on the digestive system. Prepare concentrated infusions using 1 1/2 oz of herb per quart of water.

❧ Complexion Problems

Like your hair and nails, your complexion is an indicator of your general state of health, so it isn't a good idea to use surface remedies to try and improve your complexion. They do nothing to cure the underlying problem. Treating your body as a unified whole is a better approach.

Start by applying some fresh carrot or orange juice to the skin on your face twice a week. Then follow the guidelines below.

Nutrition

Generally speaking, it's best not to eat too much meat. Here is a list of foods that can help restore or improve your complexion: grated beets or carrots seasoned with pure olive oil and lemon, cabbage, watercress, spinach, chicory, lettuce, radish, onion, olive, grapes, strawberries, dried figs, prunes, lentils, calves liver, milk, and dairy products.

Plant Power

If your complexion is not so peaches and creamy as you'd like it to be, add some of these plant remedies to your other dietary changes.

Burdock is a depurative and antiseptic recommended for all types of skin disorders. Boil 1 oz of roots in a quart of water for a few minutes, and drink three cups a day.

Nettle is an excellent depurative that will be sure to enhance your complexion. Boil 1 oz of leaves in a quart of water for a few minutes, and drink three or four cups a day.

WHAT WE LEARNED FROM MICHAEL JACKSON

Even though one or two out of every 100 people suffer from vitiligo, most of us had never heard of it until Michael Jackson announced that he was a victim. It's a condition that breaks down pigment in the skin and causes unsightly white patches to appear, usually in the same place on both sides of the body. Vitiligo is usually harmless physically, but as MJ showed us, it can be devastating psychologically. It's been around for thousands of years, but only recently have we come to recognize that it's an autoimmune disease.

Although conventional medicine doesn't offer much in the way of treatment, here are a couple of tips from the world of plants you might want to try.

- **Beet it.** Apply beet cataplasms to areas of lighter skin: Wash the leaves, crush them in a mortar and pestle, and add a little sweet almond oil.
- **Soak with cypress.** Cypress can be used to bathe the hands: Boil 1 oz of crushed berries in a half pint of water for 15 minutes and wash your hands in the decoction.

THE SKINNY ON SKIN SPOTS

There are many types of skin spots. Some may be present at birth, others develop later on in life. Most are harmless, but a few need to be looked at by a doctor.

- **Beauty spots** are usually benign and need not be treated unless they are subject to frequent irritation and start to increase in size or appear in areas that are considered unaesthetic.
- **Brown or gray areas** of skin sometimes appear on the faces of women who are in their third or fourth month of pregnancy. They generally disappear after the mother gives birth.
- **Freckles** appear on fair skin and are benign. Exposure to the sun tends to accentuate them.
- **Liver spots** are brown areas that generally appear on elderly people, especially on the backs of the hands, and have nothing to do with the liver. Although they can be surgically removed, they are not harmful.
- **Black or dark brown spots** or moles should be looked at by a doctor, especially if they're bigger around than a pencil eraser, have uneven or notched borders, have other colors in them (red, blue, white), bleed, or look unusual in any other way. These may be melanomas, which are a dangerous form of skin cancer.

For benign conditions, the remedies below can help erase unsightly skin spots.

- **Almond** helps get rid of freckles: Use bitter almond paste, or mix some almond flour with rose water and apply regularly.
- **Lily** helps eliminate various types of skin spots. Infuse 100 grams in half a liter of boiled water for a few hours, then apply locally.
- **Wild daisy** can help eliminate unsightly beauty spots: Buy some tincture, available in herbal and health food stores and some pharmacies, and use a glass applicator to put a drop on the spots you want to get rid of; repeat daily.
- **Horseradish** fades freckles: Mix a teaspoon of grated horseradish with a small amount of milk or yogurt; let stand for half an hour, then filter and apply; leave in place long enough to dry, then rinse with hot water.
- **Marigold** helps eliminate beauty and liver spots: Apply fresh marigold juice to affected areas a number of times a day. To obtain your juice, simply put some stems and flowers through a blender or extractor. Expect to wait some time before seeing results.

≫ Constipation

Constipation simply means that you have difficulty moving your bowels or that you don't do it very frequently. Most of us have gone through it at least once in our lives. Usually, it amounts to nothing more than a temporary annoyance.

While occasional constipation is not dangerous, however, a chronic inability to eliminate waste results in an accumulation of toxins in the body, and can lead to more serious health problems, including various skin disorders.

Causes of constipation vary. Nutrition is obviously important, as are psychological factors: Persons often become constipated when their day-to-day routine is disturbed, for example while traveling or living through periods of stress or emotional trauma. An agitated lifestyle, lack of physical exercise, and a diet that contains too much meat and too few vegetables also tends to cause constipation.

In some cases, persons may think they are suffering from constipation, although the real problem is related to some intestinal problem, such as an obstruction.

General Care

Although laxatives may be an effective short-term solution, becoming dependent on them will only make the problem worse. Try to use laxatives as infrequently as possible.

Lifestyle

Make sure you exercise enough. Don't let a day pass without getting out and taking a walk in the fresh air, if only for a few minutes before going to bed at night.

Nutrition

As a general rule, a diet rich in green vegetables and fruit is best. These should be accompanied by bran and whole grains (cooked oat or wheat cereal), and whole grain bread (unless you are suffering from colitis). Drink some pure spring water every morning before breakfast.

It's best to avoid laxatives as much as possible. Instead, eat prunes or soak some dried figs in water overnight and have them for breakfast. Using a couple of teaspoons of olive oil, castor oil, or honey as a spread on toast in the morning is also helpful, as are stomach massages. If you continue to suffer from chronic constipation despite these measures, consult a doctor.

Plant Power

Plants can be extremely useful in returning sluggish bowel habits to regularity. Here are some to try.

Buckthorn acts as a laxative or purgative, depending on how much you take, and will not irritate your intestines. Boil a pinch of bark in a cup of water for half an hour; add a pinch of aniseed, then let soak for five or six hours.

Chicory is both a tonic for the nervous system and a mild laxative. It helps clean the blood and improves the quality of skin that has suffered because of chronic constipation. It also acts as an intestinal antiseptic and stimulates liver functions. You can eat fresh chicory, added to salads. To prepare infusions, use 1 oz of fresh or dried (not roasted) roots per quart of boiling water. Take as needed.

Couchgrass (also called doggrass) helps eliminate urine and acts as a laxative, antiseptic, antibiotic, and mild sedative. Boil 1 oz of roots in 2/3 cup of water for one minute; discard this water, crush the softened roots, and boil them a second time in 1 1/4 quarts of water until only 1 quart remains; add 1/3 oz of licorice, zest of lemon, and sweeten with honey.

For an herbal tea that fights constipation: Mix the following ingredients: 1/3 oz of couchgrass, 1/3 oz of aniseed, 1/3 oz of buckthorn, 1/3 oz of chicory, and 1/3 oz of marshmallow. Boil the mixture for 20 minutes in 2 quarts of water; drink a cup before and after your evening meal.

❧ Convulsions

Aside from epileptic convulsions, which represent a case apart, persons most likely to experience convulsions are children running a fever of more than 102 degrees Fahrenheit. Although spectacular, the disorder rarely has serious consequences. Doctors will usually prescribe an anticonvulsive medication.

Plant Power

Convulsions need to be dealt with quickly, and the quick treatment of acute conditions generally falls within the realm of conventional medicine. The role of plants in therapy should be auxiliary. Here are two you can try.

Chickweed is a tonic. Drinking a few cups of chickweed infusion can put an end to mild convulsions. Use 1/3 oz of dried leaves per quart of boiling water and take as needed.

Valerian is a sedative and antispasmodic. Make sure not to exceed the recommended dosage—if you do, the effect can be reversed and you may become more agitated. To prepare infusions, use 1 oz of roots per quart of boiling water; remove from heat and let stand for 15 minutes. Drink a cup between meals (adults can drink up to half a quart per day).

☙ Coughing

A cough can be an unpleasant symptom, but it's actually beneficial. It helps decongest blocked breathing passages and expel toxins in phlegm. For that reason, it's not always a good idea to suppress a cough with medication.

There are many kinds of coughs, and each is an indicator of a specific type of health problem. Whooping cough, for example, is characterized by frequent hoarse coughing and a wheezing sound in the chest. Laryngitis causes hoarse coughing as mucous backs up in the throat and irritates the larynx.

Infants may cough because they are teething, while coughing in toddlers and older children may signal the presence of intestinal parasites. Coughing in adults can be a symptom of a cardiac or nervous disorder.

Plant Power

Coughing is a symptom that seems particularly responsive to plant therapy. Here are a few botanical remedies you can try at home.

Onions can help quiet coughing and encourage the airways to clear themselves of phlegm. They are also rich in Vitamin C, which is beneficial for cases of persistent cough and irritation of the breathing passages. They're most effective when cooked.

Angelica helps alleviate smoker's cough. Boil 1 1/2 oz of the plant in a quart of water for 10 minutes. Drink a cup in the morning before breakfast, and another in the evening before going to bed.

Mullein soothes a cough and helps eliminate mucous. Use 1 oz per quart of water to prepare infusions; filter through a fine cloth to remove filaments that can irritate the throat, and drink three or four cups a day.

Borage soothes irritated respiratory passages and alleviates coughing. It's recommended for cases of bronchitis and dry coughing. Infuse 1 oz in a quart of water, filter through a fine cloth to remove filaments that can irritate the throat, and drink three or four cups a day.

Maidenhair fern is recommended for cases of persistent coughing. Boil 1/2 to 1 oz of the plant in a quart of water for four minutes, and drink two cups a day.

Eucalyptus stimulates phlegm production, has an antiseptic effect on breathing passages, and calms coughing fits. Infuse 1 oz in a quart of water for 20 minutes; add a little natural honey and lemon juice, and drink four to six cups a day. You can also prepare your own eucalyptus syrup: Add 2 oz of leaves to a quart of boiling water; remove from heat and let stand overnight; filter, add 800 grams of sugar, and boil again until the liquid acquires the consistency of thick syrup; take a couple of teaspoons a few times a day.

Marshmallow soothes irritated respiratory passages and alleviates coughing. To prepare marshmallow cough syrup, soak 2 oz of marshmallow root in a quart of cold water overnight; add 1 1/2 to 2 lbs of sugar and simmer for 15 or 20 minutes.

Lavender controls coughing that brings up a lot of mucous, and has an antiseptic effect on breathing passages. Infuse 1 oz in a quart of boiled water and drink three or four cups a day.

Ground ivy helps you to expel mucous when you cough, and soothes irritated membranes in the breathing passages. It's not recommended for dry cough, though. Infuse 1 oz of flower tops in a quart of boiled water and drink two or three cups a day.

Rosemary helps quiet a cough. Drink a cup of infusion after meals: Use 1/2 oz of plant per quart of boiled water.

Wild thyme works well to ease persistent or chronic coughing. Infuse 1 oz in a quart of boiled water and drink three cups a day. Cultivated thyme helps tame convulsive coughing. Infuse 1 oz of the plant in a quart of hot water (do not boil) and drink three or four cups a day.

Coltsfoot is an excellent remedy for persistent harsh coughing accompanied by expectoration of phlegm, spasms, and bronchitis. Drink a few cups of infusion, sweetened with natural honey, or a little aniseed, during the course of the day; use 1 oz per quart of boiled water to prepare infusions. To prepare coltsfoot syrup, mix 1 oz each of coltsfoot, hyssop, and plantain with 2/3 oz of malva and a pinch of red poppy flowers; pour a quart of boiling water over the mixture, cover and let stand overnight Filter the brew and add about a kilogram of sugar; heat in a double boiler until the liquid acquires the consistency of syrup. This remedy cannot be stored for long periods of time.

Speedwell helps expel mucous and acts as a tonic that rebuilds strength after persistent coughing. Use 1 oz of plant per quart of boiled water to prepare infusions. Drink a cup before meals and before going to bed at night.

You can also make an herbal mixture, comprising 1/3 oz of borage and a pinch each of fumitory, red poppy, rosemary, and eucalyptus; infuse in a quart of boiled water for a few minutes, and drink a few cups during the course of the day.

✎ Cuts and Scrapes

The sooner you treat a cut or scrape, the better. The longer it remains untended, the higher your risk of infection—a complication that can lead to real trouble.

Before you do anything else, you'll need to stop any bleeding and disinfect the wound properly with hydrogen peroxide or an antibiotic cream (both available at your local drugstore). If you think a cut is large or deep enough to require stitches, call your doctor or go to the emergency room at your community hospital.

Plant Power

Once the cut is clean, you can use herbs both internally and externally to help the healing process. Here are some to try.

NATURAL DISINFECTANTS

People who always head to the store to buy disinfectants—either for cuts and scrapes or for surfaces in the home—may be interested to know that a number of completely natural substances exist that are just as effective and much less toxic to the respiratory system and skin. Here are three of the best:

- **Eucalyptus** is an antiseptic that helps prevent infection. The tincture can be used instead of iodine to disinfect minor cuts and burns and accelerate healing. Eucalyptus vapor disinfects sickrooms and eliminates bacteria, while inhaling the vapor opens respiratory passages. Boil 1/2 oz of leaves per quart of water in an open pot to fumigate rooms or prepare inhalations.
- **Pine** is a disinfectant that also promotes healing. Boil 1 oz of cones in a quart of water for five minutes, and use the vapor as an inhalation or to fumigate sickrooms.
- **Vinegar:** Use this mixture to prepare a powerful disinfectant cleaner for floors, sinks, toilets, bathtubs, bedstands, pots and pans, and sick-rooms. It will get rid of musty odors and leave floors, walls, and bathrooms sparkling. Soak the following plants in 2 1/2 quarts of cider vinegar for 10 days, either in direct sunlight or near some other heat source: a pinch of sweet flag, a pinch of cinnamon, a pinch of cloves, a pinch of nutmeg, 1 oz of wormwood, 1 oz of absinthe, 1 oz of lavender, 1 oz of rosemary, and 1 oz of sage. Filter, press well, and add a few cloves of garlic. Filter again a few days later and store in a sealed container. For external use on your body, dilute a small amount of the mixture in four times its volume of water. This disinfectant can also be used internally, as a preventive measure against epidemics of contagious disease: Drink one teaspoon, diluted in a glass of water, every hour until the danger has passed.

Aloe vera was known even in the time of Alexander the Great to have amazing curative powers. These days, we believe it prevents infection and greatly accelerates healing of cuts and burns. Aloe vera is best used fresh, and because it's easy to grow indoors, why not keep one around just in case? To treat open cuts or wounds, simply cut off a lower leaf and squeeze the pulp directly onto the cut after you've disinfected it. You can also buy pure aloe vera gel in some pharmacies and most health food stores. Soak some gauze in the gel and apply directly to the wound to promote coagulation and healing.

Goldenseal helps heal wounds and reduces the risk of infection. To prepare your own goldenseal ointment, mix equal parts of goldenseal and
American red elm with a little water to form a paste. You can also mix goldenseal with a plantain ointment.

St. John's wort has long been used to make St. John's oil, a very effective traditional remedy for cuts and burns. It's a good idea to prepare your
oil in advance, in case of an emergency. Fill a glass container with St. John's
wort, then cover it with extra virgin olive oil. Seal the container and let it
stand in direct sunlight, or near a heat source, for five or six weeks, shaking
or stirring the mixture from time to time. Filter and store in an opaque container (the oil can be kept for up to two years). Use as an external application on open cuts, wounds, and bruises.

Butterburr is effective for treating infected cuts: Wash some fresh leaves
and apply them directly to the wound. Cover the leaves with some gauze to
keep them in place; change the dressing a few times a day.

Yarrow helps heal cuts. Buy some yarrow tincture at your local health
food store, herbal store, or pharmacy, and mix with nine parts water. To
stop a nosebleed, soak a cotton swab in the mixture and place in the bleeding nostril. Yarrow infusions, applied locally, help heal purulent or infected
wounds or abscesses and reduce swelling. Prepare infusions using 1 oz of
plant per quart of water. Yarrow sap can also be applied directly to cuts:
Rinse some fresh leaves, then crush with a rolling pin and place on the
affected area.

Cabbage accelerates healing and helps alleviate pain. Wash a few cabbage
leaves, remove the outer edges and flatten them with a rolling pin; soak the
leaves in some boric acid for a few hours, and then apply them directly to the
affected area, using a bandage to hold them in place. Change the compress
twice a day.

Lavender is an antiseptic that promotes healing. Use decoctions (1 oz per
quart of water) or lavender oil: Soak a handful of flowers in a quart of olive
oil for three days in direct sunlight, or near some other heat source; filter and
repeat until the oil smells very strongly of lavender. You can also soak 1/3 cup
of lavender, 2 oz of St. John's wort flower tops and 1 oz of chamomile in half
a quart of 90-proof alcohol for 15 days. Filter the mixture and add a pinch
of camphor and a third of a quart of water; shake well before use.

Lily accelerates healing of superficial cuts. Soak a handful of petals in some brandy, then apply the pulp to affected areas.

Savory is an antiseptic that can be used to treat cuts and wounds, as well as throat and mouth infections. To prepare infusions, add 1 oz of the plant to a quart of boiled water.

Sage is an antiseptic that accelerates the healing of cuts and wounds. Dip compresses in a sage infusion: 2 oz of leaves per quart of water. Adding a little vinegar makes the remedy more effective.

Marigold is an antiseptic that combats inflammation and accelerates healing. Use decoctions or tinctures, both available in health food and herbal stores. Dilute a teaspoon of tincture in three teaspoons of boiled water.

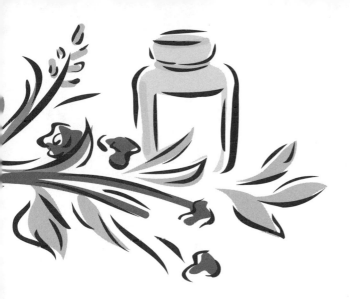

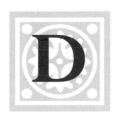

❧ Dental Problems

Two things make a great smile: sparkling eyes and beautiful teeth. Sparkling eyes reflect joy from within. Beautiful teeth reflect proper dental care. We don't intend to provide an exhaustive description here of how you should care for your teeth, but we will give you one reminder: Dental hygiene is, first and foremost, a matter of prevention. Because decayed tooth enamel doesn't grow back, the state of your teeth as you get older depends, to a great extent, on how you treat them while you're young.

Nutrition

Everyone knows that refined sugar causes tooth decay, but a growing body of research seems to indicate that refined flour is also responsible for weakening teeth.

Eating raw crunchy vegetables, on the other hand, helps keep teeth strong, and allows you to absorb more nutrients, because high temperatures destroy at least part of the nutritional value of most foods.

Eating calcium-rich foods like cheese, walnuts, soy, almonds, dried beans and peas, lentils, whole grains and rice, spinach, lettuce, celery, oats, and barley prevents teeth from getting yellow.

Drinking nettle infusions helps calcium absorption. Eating crunchy raw apples also helps keep tooth enamel white and strengthens your gums.

SAVE YOUR BREATH

Many people who have bad breath are not aware of it because no one dares or cares enough to tell them. But if you've ever had to work closely with someone suffering from halitosis, you know how unpleasant it can be. The problem can become a real handicap, both professionally and personally.

Improper dental hygiene is the most common cause, so making sure that no food remains lodged between your teeth, where it will slowly rot and produce the characteristic fetid odor of halitosis, is an important preventive measure. In some cases, however, halitosis is a side effect of a liver, digestive, or bronchial problem.

Fortunately, you can get big help from three little plants if bad breath is a problem for you.

- **Dill.** Chew dill seeds to neutralize unpleasant mouth odors.
- **Mint.** Make an infusion and gargle with it several times a day.
- **Sage.** This also makes a great infusion for gargling.

General Care

Of course you should brush your teeth thoroughly morning and night. Daily flossing, which removes particles lodged between your teeth, is also a good idea, because these particles can decompose, resulting in bad breath (halitosis) and attack gums, causing irreversible retraction (periodontitis). Gum retraction of only two or three millimeters every five or six years is more than enough to result in the loosening and eventual loss of teeth. And some recent research has revealed a link between gum disease and heart disease.

Have your cavities treated by a dentist to prevent later complications. Also, see your dentist for a cleaning at least once a year, even if there is nothing obviously wrong, because removing tartar buildup is important for preventing gingivitis.

Plant Power

Here are some great botanical aids to proper dental hygiene.

Garlic has antiseptic properties that can help combat tooth or gum disease. It also helps alleviate pain. Apply freshly crushed garlic directly to the affected area.

Chamomile has a tranquilizing effect that helps soothe pain while you're waiting to see a dentist. It's especially recommended for children. Pour a cup of boiling water over 1 oz of chamomile leaves and let stand for three minutes. Use the warm leaves for local applications and the liquid as a mouthwash. Repeat the treatments several times each day.

Watercress helps strengthen gums—simply chew a few fresh watercress leaves. Watercress also makes an effective treatment for swollen gums.

Marshmallow soothes inflammation, which makes it especially useful for treating mouth abscesses. Boil 2/3 oz of marshmallow in a quart of water for 15 minutes and use the lukewarm liquid as a mouthwash several times a day.

Sage prevents gums from bleeding and teeth from loosening. Use infusions as a mouthwash: 2/3 oz of plant per quart of boiling water; let stand for 10 minutes.

Thyme can be used to make herbal toothpaste: Mix powdered thyme, powdered sage, and clay with a little water. Essence of thyme alleviates dental pain. Thyme can also be used as a rub to disinfect lesions and alleviate pain: Soak 1/3 cup of thyme in one quart of brandy for 10 days. Denture wearers can add a teaspoon to their mouthwash.

☙ Depression

Depression can affect you after a sad, disappointing, or stressful event in your life, or it can strike like a bolt from the blue, for no apparent reason and with no prior warning. We don't fully understand why this should be so, but we do know how to treat you when it happens. The treatment depends, first of all, on the type of depression you have.

Severe depression requires professional treatment, not home remedies. Symptoms may include deep hopelessness; a general lack of interest in life; loss of libido, appetite, or the ability to feel pleasure; sudden changes in weight; anxiety and irritability; or sleep disturbances.

Mild depression, or *dysthymia*, is characterized by recurring feelings of discouragement, listlessness, fatigue, apathy, and anxiety. You can feel mildly depressed because you didn't get the raise you were hoping for or because you don't have a job at all. You can get depressed from working too much or because your diet is deficient in minerals or vitamins. Chronic depression can even be caused by a heart condition.

BURNOUT

Job burnout has become too common an occurrence in the modern workplace. It's the contemporary equivalent of what was commonly called a nervous breakdown a few years ago. Strangely enough, experiencing burnout has almost become a badge of achievement these days, signaling an unquestioning dedication to work. And yet the harmful effects of burnout are far-reaching and can undermine the quality of a person's life—and productivity—for years.

The road to burnout progresses in four identifiable stages:

1. **Tunnel vision.** People first become extremely demanding of their own professional performance, and their enthusiasm makes them oblivious to anything outside of their work.

2. **Exhaustion/stagnation.** Disillusionment and dissatisfaction begin setting in, like cracks in the foundation of a building.

3. **Frustration.** This phase usually signals the onset of physical and psychological exhaustion. People tend to seek scapegoats. They become aggressive, lose control of their emotions easily, and start questioning their self-worth and the value of what they're doing.

4. **Apathy and depression.** People who reach this stage either quit what they're doing and change professions or get dragged down by feelings of impotence and worthlessness. They may resent any interference or show of authority and become cynical and blasé, or feel as if they are being victimized. Over-consumption of alcohol and medications often goes hand in hand with insomnia. Productivity drops as physical health problems like ulcers, frequent infections, and improper digestion make the situation even more intolerable.

The road back from burnout requires lots of support from loved ones, friends, and even professional therapists. But the world of plants also has a few remedies to offer. Try using ginseng, as you would for depression, or give these herbs a chance:

- **Maté**, native to South America, is an excellent tonic that combats fatigue and stimulates the heart and nervous system. Rich in Vitamin C and chlorophyll, maté improves intellectual functions and physical endurance and helps eliminate toxins. Use a few leaves per cup of boiled water. You can drink as much as you like, for as long as you like.

- **Rosemary** is a stimulant recommended for cases of general weakness and physical or intellectual fatigue. Persons who have digestive problems should not use this plant too often. Infuse 1 oz of flower tops in a quart of boiled water for 20 minutes, and drink three to five cups a day.

- **Sage** is an excellent tonic and stimulant for the nervous system. Infusions require 1/2 oz of plant per quart of boiled water. Drink three cups a day.

Plant Power

Although the medicinal plants mentioned below could help get you through a difficult period, you should not rely solely on herbal remedies to recharge your batteries and restore the energy you seem to be lacking. Exercise, a healthy diet, and attending to stressful areas in your life are important weapons in your arsenal for fighting depression.

Asian ginseng increases resistance to stress, improves concentration, and raises your energy level. Persons who have been suffering from mild depression for an extended period should ingest about 500 mg (one capsule) of dried ginseng root daily for 10 days and repeat the cure every two months. Younger, more active persons should not take ginseng for more than three weeks at a time.

Mistletoe is an excellent remedy for fatigue (it also happens to be a lot less expensive than ginseng), especially if your condition is associated with cardiac problems or slow metabolism. Mistletoe regulates circulation and heart functions, and is often prescribed as a cure for both hypertension (high blood pressure) and hypotension (low blood pressure). Mistletoe is prepared cold: Soak a teaspoon of twigs in a cup of cold water for 24 hours. Drink one cup per day, in three equal portions, morning, noon, and night. If you can obtain fresh mistletoe leaves, soak six teaspoons in 1 1/2 cups of cold water for eight hours, and drink a mouthful at frequent intervals during the day.

✑ Dermatitis

Dermatitis is a catch-all word that describes many types of skin irritations from many causes. Dermatitis can result from allergic reactions, bug bites, viruses, chemical irritants (such as those found in common household cleaners), acne, eczema, scabies, impetigo, psoriasis, and extreme temperatures. In some cases, even the homeopathic remedy Rhus Toxicodendron can have an adverse effect on the skin.

Conventional medications can also cause problems when taken in large doses or for extended periods of time. Analgesics, barbiturates, bromides, cortisone-based medications, laxatives, quinine, sulfa drugs, and medications containing mercury can all cause reactions in the skin.

TOP 10 FOODS TO AVOID IF YOU HAVE DERMATITIS

Stay away from canned, smoked, salted, marinated, fried, or fat meats like sausages, blood pudding, sweetbreads, brains, tripe, pigs feet, etc. Also avoid fried, salted, smoked, dried, or canned fish (including sardines). Don't eat black beans or sorrel, greasy soups or stews, peanut butter, pastries, candies, soft drinks, and fried foods in general (at least not often).

General Care

You cannot limit the treatment of dermatitis to external local applications. A more systemic approach is necessary, one that includes lots of fresh air and exercise, juice, water, herbal cures, relaxation, and other stress-reducing techniques, as well as depurative and diuretic medicinal plants that stimulate kidney functions and clean the blood. Bathing affected areas in hot milk curd can also be helpful in certain cases.

Nutrition

Like every other organ in your body, your skin is profoundly sensitive to the foods you eat. By making some simple dietary changes, you can go a long way toward maintaining a fresh, healthy complexion. Here's what to do.

Make your diet natural. Avoid industrially processed, refined foods. Many of the chemicals added to them can wreak havoc with your skin.

Add some Bs. B-complex vitamins can help by reducing stress: Brewer's yeast, which contains all the B vitamins and is very rich in Vitamin B8, can be effective for combating certain types of dermatitis.

Go with grains. Wheat germ is another excellent food supplement for persons with skin problems like eczema or acne.

Stop at the salad bar. Salads containing organically grown nettle or spinach sprouts help eliminate eczema rashes and pimples.

Avoid acids. When impaired liver functions are part of the problem, as is often the case, avoid acidic foods: lemons, oranges, grapefruit, berries, raw apples, wine, cider, coffee, chocolate, and cocoa.

STOP THAT ITCH!

Pruritis, the medical term for itching, is not a disease but a symptom, signaling the presence of a health problem that may be serious or benign. Aside from insect bites, itching can be a symptom of diabetes, arthritis, constipation, gout, menopause, scabies, intestinal parasites, eczema, hives, psoriasis, industrial diseases caused by exposure to various irritants, or even cancer.

For cases of temporary itching, apply vinegar diluted in a little hot water, or some fresh leek juice if you don't have any of the plants recommended below. You can also massage affected areas with a slice of raw potato or some grated raw potato. Also, try replacing your usual soap with one that has an acidic pH. If none of this helps, here are some plant teas to try.

- **Beet leaves** help alleviate itching: Boil 2 oz of fresh chopped leaves in a quart of water for 10 minutes; drink two cups per day, and use the decoction for local applications.
- **Cabbage** is very effective as an external application: Boil 200 grams of leaves in a quart of water for 20 minutes and use the softened leaves as compresses or to bathe affected areas.
- **Mint** helps alleviate itching: Prepare infusions using 2 oz of leaves per quart of water and bathe affected areas.
- **Dandelion** eliminates itching caused by skin disorders: Simply chew 5 or 10 dandelion stems, picked while the plant is flowering.
- **Purple loosestrife** compresses alleviate itching and vaginal pruritis. Boil 2 oz of flower tops in a quart of water for 10 minutes.
- **Speedwell** is recommended for elderly persons who suffer from chronic pruritis because of its depurative effect. For internal use infuse 1 oz of flower tops in a quart of water. For external use boil 2 oz of flowering plant in a quart of water for five to 10 minutes.

Plant Power

Keeping your skin healthy and beautiful is an area where botanical remedies can really do a great job. Here are some suggestions.

Artichoke acts as a diuretic and helps eliminate bile. It's recommended for cases of acne and eczema related to liver problems or high cholesterol. To prepare decoctions, boil 1 oz of leaves in a quart of water for 10 minutes.

Burdock is one of the best plants for treating skin problems, notably acne and eczema. Its depurative, diuretic, and laxative properties help eliminate toxins. Drink a cup of infusion in the morning before breakfast, and one or two more during the course of the day.

Chamomile soothes sensitive, irritated, dry or itching skin. Infuse 2 oz of chamomile in two cups of boiling water for 10 minutes Use cotton balls to bathe affected areas with the liquid, then soak a piece of linen in the chamomile infusion and apply directly to the skin. Leave it in place for 10 minutes. Repeat the treatment morning and evening for a week.

Carrots can be used to make compresses for the treatment of facial dermatitis. Grate some fresh carrot and apply directly to affected areas of skin.

Celandine ointment helps eliminate psoriasis crusts. Use an extractor to obtain a pinch of pure celandine juice, then mix with 2 oz of lard. Keep the ointment refrigerated. Apply twice a day.

Chervil is a digestive, diuretic, and stimulant that makes an effective remedy for eczema and other skin problems. You can combine chervil with yarrow and dandelion to prepare infusions.

Chicory purifies the blood, improves your complexion, and helps eliminate skin problems. Drink infusions: 1 oz of leaves (not roots) per quart of boiling water.

Couchgrass (or doggrass) is a diuretic and depurative that helps eliminate bile. Use it to treat eczema: Boil 1 oz of root stalks in a cup of water for one minute; discard the water, crush the plant, and boil again in 1 1/4 quarts of water until a cup has evaporated. Add some zest of lemon, filter, and cool. You can drink up to a quart per day.

Watercress juice is a depurative that is very rich in vitamins and minerals. Drink half a cup of fresh juice every day. To increase its effectiveness, combine watercress with a lettuce decoction (boil 2 oz of lettuce in a quart of water for 20 minutes), chicory infusion (see above), and fumitory infusions (see below). Watercress also helps eliminate red splotches caused by exposure to sunlight: Bathe affected areas with 2 oz of watercress juice mixed with two teaspoons of essence of bitter almond.

Bittersweet compresses are recommended for treating pityriasis (dry scaly dermatitis) and herpes. Prepare decoctions and apply as a lotion: Boil 1 oz of roots in a quart of water for 30 minutes.

Fumitory is a depurative that effectively combats pityriasis (dry, scaly dermatitis) and other skin problems. It also regulates secretions of bile. To prepare infusions use 1 oz of the plant per quart of boiling water, and drink two or three cups a day (you'll have to get used to the bitter taste).

Marshmallow and malva make poultices that soothe irritation and inflammation. You can also apply freshly pressed juice to affected areas to eliminate psoriasis crusts. Prepare poultices with the leaves of either plant and apply directly to affected areas. For psoriasis and dermatitis related to nervous tension, soak 6 1⁄2 oz of either plant in some water overnight and add to your bath water (keep your chest above water while taking your bath).

Mint helps heal tissues and soothes inflammation and itching. Use it to treat eczema, scabies, and other types of dermatitis. Infuse 2 oz of leaves in a quart of boiled water for 10 minutes and use the liquid to prepare compresses. You can prepare some mint oil: Place 2 oz of fresh mint in 1 1⁄2 quarts of pure olive oil; let stand in direct sunlight or near some other heat source for a week; filter and store in a sealed container; apply directly to affected areas.

Walnut soothes pain and itching caused by dermatitis. Apply freshly crushed or boiled leaves directly to affected areas.

Nettle is a diuretic and depurative that purifies the blood, helps eliminate bile, and detoxifies your organism. It is especially recommended for treating chronic eczema and hives. Boil a tablespoon of leaves or roots in a cup of water (two minutes for leaves, five minutes for roots); remove from heat and let stand for five minutes; drink one or two cups each day. You can also add fresh nettle to salads.

Wild pansy is another plant that is very effective for treating skin problems. Its depurative, diuretic, and laxative properties help combat a wide range of skin-related disorders, including milk crust (impetigo), hives, herpes, psoriasis, acne, and eczema. It is especially recommended for children. Drink infusions or add fresh leaves to salads. (When used to treat acne, wild pansy will initially cause pimples to form as the plant re-balances your organic functions. Don't worry, the eruptions will soon fade and disappear completely.) Drink two or three cups a day, one in the morning before breakfast and one before your evening meal.

Dandelion is a diuretic and helps in the treatment of dermatitis associated with a liver insufficiency. Boil 1 oz to 2 oz of roots in a quart of water for half an hour, remove from heat, and let stand for four hours. Drink two cups a day, between meals.

Plantain is a mild astringent that accelerates the healing of minor skin lesions. Apply fresh sap directly to affected areas, or drink decoctions: Boil 3 1/2 oz of leaves in a quart of water for 20 minutes.

Marigold is recommended for the treatment of various skin disorders, including fungal dermatitis, milk crust, impetigo, eczema, boils, warts, and acne. Boil 3 oz of leaves or 2 oz of flowers in a quart of water for 10 minutes, and drink two cups a day. Marigold ointment helps combat fungal infections on the feet. Boil 3 oz of petals in half a quart of water for 45 minutes; filter, and add an equal weight of lard; then simmer until all the liquid has evaporated. The same ointment can be used to treat vaginal fungal infections.

Speedwell can be used to treat chronic eczema, as well as other skin disorders. Wash stems and flowers thoroughly, then put them through a juice extractor. Store the juice in your fridge. Take two or three teaspoons a day, mixed with nettle infusion.

➥ Diabetes

If you are frequently thirsty or hungry, if the volume of your urine increases significantly, if you suffer from constant itching, if cuts—even minor ones—don't seem to heal, and if you begin to develop various skin problems such as boils or eczema, then you might be suffering from diabetes. The only way to find out for sure is to consult a doctor.

Having diabetes means you have too much sugar (glucose) in your blood. That can affect everything from your energy level to the health of your heart, eyes, and nervous system.

There are two main types of diabetes. Type 1, insulin dependent diabetes, occurs when your pancreas can no longer make insulin, the chemical that allows your cells to absorb sugar and turn it into energy. Most people with this form of the disease take daily injections of insulin to control it. Type 2, latent diabetes, occurs when your pancreas doesn't make enough insulin, or when your cells start ignoring the insulin that you make. Diet and exercise alone can sometimes keep this form of the disease under control, although some people will also need to take supplemental insulin.

Nutrition

Generally speaking, persons suffering from diabetes should reduce their consumption of starches and sugars, animal and vegetable fats, and proteins (meat, eggs, and cheese). It's also best to stop drinking alcohol.

Here are some other dietary changes you can make that will help keep your blood sugar under control.

Munch mushrooms. They contain a sugar-reducing substance.

Snack on raw vegetables.
Carrot juice, salads containing endive and onions, and cold, first-pressed sunflower seed oil are especially recommended.

Enjoy an artichoke. This vegetable, which actually contains insulin, represents one carbohydrate that can be easily assimilated by diabetics. Garlic, fenugreek, coconut, spinach, and leeks also help regulate sugar levels in the blood. Celery and cucumber juice are recommended for the same reason.

Supplement with brewer's yeast. It increases diabetics' tolerance for sugars that are stored in the liver and helps eliminate skin problems characteristic of the disorder. Take brewer's yeast supplements daily.

Plant Power

Although nature offers us a variety of sugar-reducing substances, you should never ignore your doctor's instructions in the hope that plants alone

---

THE WARNING SIGNS OF DIABETES

The American Diabetes Association estimates that 16 million Americans have diabetes, but a third of them don't know it! You don't have to be in the dark. Here are the ways in which diabetes announces itself. If you have any of these symptoms, see a doctor as soon as you can.

- You've lost weight without trying.
- You have to urinate a lot.
- You often feel very hungry.
- You often feel very thirsty.
- You sometimes have blurry vision.
- You often feel tired.
- You have frequent, persistent headaches.
- You have dry, itchy skin.

can cure your condition. They can, however, greatly contribute to your good health if you're dealing with diabetes. Here are some to try.

Burdock helps lower blood sugar levels and also combats skin problems associated with diabetes. Boil 2 oz of roots in a quart of water for 10 minutes; drink a cup in the morning before breakfast, and one or two more during the course of the day.

Chicory makes a mildly laxative infusion, which has a tonic effect on the liver and intestines, regulates blood sugar levels, reduces the volume of urine, and slakes thirst. To prepare infusions, use 2 oz of dried roots or 1/2 oz of dried leaves per quart of boiling water. Drink a cup before meals. You can also add chicory leaves to salads.

Eucalyptus helps lower sugar levels in the blood and urine and is also a stimulant and antiseptic for the urinary tract. Prepare infusions using 1 oz of leaves per quart of water, and drink four or five cups a day.

Goat's rue lowers blood sugar levels and increases tolerance for carbohydrates. Regular testing is essential, however, in order to ensure that you don't ingest too many carbohydrates and run the risk of falling into a diabetic coma. Prepare infusions using 2/3 oz of plant per quart of boiling water, and drink three or four cups a day.

Green or yellow string beans reduce blood sugar levels and are helpful in controlling mild cases of diabetes. For maximum effect, beans should be harvested before they reach full maturity and ingested along with a nettle or berry infusion.

Mulberries and blackberries have long been used as a remedy for diabetes and can reduce, or even cure, high sugar concentrations in the urine. Prepare infusions using 2 oz of leaves per quart of boiling water, and drink three cups a day before meals. You can also buy a commercially prepared extract at health food and herbal stores, and some pharmacies.

Blueberry extract is so effective for reducing blood sugar levels that it has been nicknamed vegetal insulin. Leaves should be harvested before the plant reaches full maturity and mixed with equal parts of green beans, nettle, or dandelion for maximum effectiveness. To prepare infusions, use a handful of leaves per quart of boiling water, and drink the whole amount during the course of the day. You can also soak the leaves in two quarts of cold water overnight and then boil off half the water.

Walnut reduces blood sugar levels, and alleviates thirst and the need to urinate. Prepare infusions using 2/3 oz of leaves per quart of boiling water, and drink throughout the day.

Nettle not only lowers blood sugar levels, but also acts as a depurative and disinfectant; combats eczema, allergic rashes, and diarrhea; and helps restore vigor in persons suffering from general fatigue. Boil 1 1/2 oz of roots in a quart of water for five minutes (two minutes if you use leaves), remove the brew from the heat, and let stand for 10 minutes Drink three or four cups a day.

Dandelion can be used to treat diabetes, as well as various skin disorders. Plants should be harvested before they produce flowers, as they are much less bitter. If you pick your own, make sure you pick them well away from roads and houses to avoid getting contaminated plants. Chew about a dozen stems a day, and add leaves to salads twice a day. To prepare decoctions, chop up 2 oz of roots and boil in a quart of water for 10 minutes. Drink a number of cups during the course of the day. To prepare infusions, use about 2 oz of fresh or dried leaves per quart of boiling water.

✍ Diarrhea

We've all had it, and we all hate it. Its causes range from stress and overly rich food to more serious problems, such as gastroenteritis, food poisoning, dysentery, food allergies, colitis, kidney disorders, and a host of other diseases. It can come and go quickly, or it can last for days. It can make you feel crampy, grumpy, and sore, and it can chain you to the bathroom like a puppy on a leash.

Yet, as miserable as it can make you, diarrhea can be useful because it helps clean out your digestive system, so sometimes you're better off letting it run its course. It's when the condition persists for an overly long period, which can make you dehydrated, that steps should be taken to remedy the situation.

If diarrhea is accompanied by persistent high fever, consult a doctor. You may have dysentery, symptoms of which include abdominal pain, fever, and general weight loss. Because plants can play only a secondary role in curing dysentery, seeing a doctor for an antibiotic prescription is recommended.

IF YOUR BABY HAS WATERY BOWEL MOVEMENTS

Infants, with their developing digestive systems, seem especially vulnerable to bouts of diarrhea. To treat diarrhea in infants, use the following recipe for three days: Boil equal amounts of coarse, freshly ground wheat, barley, and oats; let stand for a few minutes, then boil again until reduced by a third; filter and feed while still warm. But beware: Diarrhea in infants can sometimes be a sign of an ear infection, so if your baby has a fever, take him or her to a doctor.

As a general rule, all other cases of severe or bloody diarrhea should come under a doctor's care as well.

In cases that cause severe rectal soreness, take sitz baths in very cold water.

Nutrition

Obviously, nutrition plays a crucial role in preventing and curing digestive disorders. When you're fighting diarrhea, try to avoid the following foods: rhubarb, milk, bread, sauces containing large amounts of fat, and anything that tends to cause intestinal fermentation, such as fruit, raw vegetables, sweets, and raw or cooked cabbage. Instead, opt for mild cheeses, oats, potatoes, natural rice, and astringent fruits like apples and bananas.

Plant Power

Agrimony is a flowering shrub that contains tannin, a substance that combats diarrhea, enteritis, and chronic liver disorders. Boil 1 oz of leaves for five minutes; remove from heat and let stand for 10 minutes. Drink three cups a day, between meals.

Fresh wild garlic makes an effective treatment for both acute and chronic diarrhea. Add it to salads, soups, or vegetable dishes. You can also prepare a liquor: Fill a glass container with finely chopped, fresh cloves or leaves and cover them with 40-proof alcohol; seal the container and let it stand in direct sunlight or near a heat source for two weeks. Take 15 drops a day, diluted in a glass of water.

Ladies mantle acts as an astringent on inflamed mucous membranes, which means it can help combat nonbacterial diarrhea. Drink two or three tablespoons of ladies mantle decoction per day: boil a pinch of leaves in 1/3 of a cup of water for 10 minutes.

Bistort is a gorgeous white flower that helps alleviate diarrhea because of its high starch and tannin content. Soak a pinch of ground or chopped roots in 1/3 of a cup of water for 15 minutes, then drink; repeat twice a day.

Carrot juice helps combat infant diarrhea, but in adults, it's more effective for treating constipation.

Carob is also helpful for treating infant diarrhea. Fill a bottle with a carob decoction: Boil 2 oz of carob flour in a quart of water for 10 minutes (for infants under six months old) or in 1/3 of a cup of water (for infants more than six months old).

WHEN DIARRHEA ISN'T JUST DIARRHEA

Caused by bacteria or parasites, dysentery is a far worse condition than the average case of diarrhea. Often caused by tropical fruit, this disease is characterized by an ulcerous inflammation of the large intestine, accompanied by colic and copious, bloody, loose stool. If you suspect you have dysentery, see a doctor as soon as possible.

Patients are generally isolated and confined to bed. A doctor will prescribe antibiotics to kill the bacteria or parasite that is causing the problem.

One effective preventive measure is to wash very thoroughly all fruits and vegetables that come from tropical countries. If you visit a tropical country, eat only fruits or vegetables that have been washed in clean water, or that can be peeled.

Blackcurrant is recommended for cases of chronic diarrhea. To prepare infusions, use 2/3 oz of young leaves per half quart of boiling water; drink four or five cups a day.

Huckleberry combats diarrhea and intestinal inflammation. Use it to prepare decoctions: Boil two cups of roots or bark in 1 1/2 quarts of water, until a third of the water has evaporated; take one or two teaspoons at a time, four or five times a day (more often if necessary).

Plantain combats diarrhea, but only when you take it in small doses. In large doses, however, the same plant acts as a laxative. Grind up 1 2/3 oz of fresh roots and 1 oz of seeds, then boil them in a quart of water until a third of the water has evaporated. Add a little sugar and bring the water to a boil one more time. Drink one or two cups a day.

Blackberry is an astringent plant that is also rich in tannin and makes an effective treatment for diarrhea, dysentery, and gastritis. Prepare decoctions by boiling 1 1/2 oz of leaves in a quart of water for two minutes; remove from heat and let stand for 10 minutes. Drink four cups a day.

✺ Dizzy Spells

Everyone knows what it's like to feel dizzy—your head spins, you can't stand or walk straight, and you feel nauseated. It's as if the earth were no longer solid beneath your feet.

Feeling a little dizzy if you're on a roller coaster ride or riding a ski lift is normal. But if you suffer from vertigo for no apparent reason, you should see a doctor as soon as you can, because dizzy spells can signal the presence of a serious health problem like high blood pressure, an ear infection, or a brain tumor.

Plant Power

Vertigo is a symptom, not a disorder. The plants listed below may alleviate vertigo temporarily, but they will not cure the underlying problem, which requires a careful diagnosis and appropriate treatment by a qualified health professional.

Hawthorn is recommended for cases of vertigo linked to nervous problems or hypertension. Infuse 1 oz of flowers in a quart of water for 10 minutes, and drink two or three cups a day.

Mistletoe acts as a tranquilizer and is an effective remedy for hypertension and other circulation problems. Use 1/2 oz per quart of water to prepare infusions and drink three or four cups a day.

Lavender is a mild sedative that can be very helpful for treating cases of vertigo. Use 1 oz per quart of water to prepare infusions. Drink three or four cups a day.

Mint is a stimulant and antispasmodic that has a tonic effect on the organism. Infuse 1 oz of leaves in a quart of water, and drink three or four cups a day.

Lemon balm (melissa) is a sedative and antispasmodic that alleviates vertigo. Infuse 1/2 oz of dried flower tops in a quart of water and drink three or four cups of infusion per day.

Sage helps strengthen persons who are convalescing from an illness or who suffer from general fatigue. Prepare infusions using 1 oz of plant per quart of water and drink three or four cups a day.

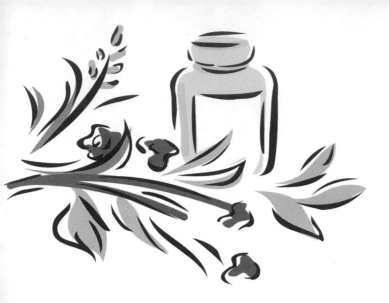

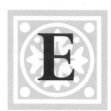

Eye Problems

Fact: If a monkey eats too many unripe bananas, the whites of its eyes will turn green (so will its tongue). Tell that to anyone who doubts that consuming botanicals can have an impact on the eye. Fortunately, using the right herbs can have a much more positive effect on the eyes of humans.

So can good circulation and adequate rest, both of which are also essential for keeping your eyes in good shape. The better your circulation, the more blood reaches your eyes, providing them with the nutrients and oxygen they need to stay healthy. And the more you rest, the more your eyes are able to recover from the stresses and strains—everything from pollution to sun glare—that assault them daily.

Nutrition

It is true that carrots, which are rich in carotene (also called pro-Vitamin A), improve vision. Lettuce contains a lot of Vitamin D, as do bananas, watercress, spinach, and tomatoes. Vitamin B2 is also effective for treating certain types of vision problems—your best natural source is brewer's yeast. Silica, an oligo-element found in horsetail, is also very good for your eyes.

Plant Power

Burdock. External application of burdock firms loose skin under the eyes. Taken internally, it has a depurative effect (cleans the blood) that helps alleviate swelling around the eyes. To prepare decoctions, boil 2 oz of powdered roots in 1 cup of water for 10 minutes; remove from heat, and infuse for 10 minutes. Drink a cup in the morning before breakfast, and apply onion poultices (see the next page).

Blueberry clears up eye inflammation and makes the pupils and whites of the eyes shine. It's also recommended for the treatment of tired, weak, or infected eyes. Bathe your eyes three times a day with compresses dipped in blueberry lotion: Mix 1 pinch of blueberry leaves, 1/3 oz of plantain leaves, and 1 pinch of sweet clover; pour 5 oz of boiling water over the mixture and continue boiling for five minutes; remove from heat and infuse for 10 minutes; filter well through a fine cloth.

Chamomile soothes fatigued eyes and alleviates swollen eyelids. It also helps cure eye infections. Apply chamomile compresses at night before going to bed. To prepare a concentrated decoction use 60 to 80 grams of plant per quart of water. To remove bags under the eyes, combine chamomile with plantain.

THE DO'S AND DON'TS OF EYE COMPRESSES

Nothing relieves tired, sore eyes like a warm compress. It's a simple, safe, and effective remedy, but there is a right way and wrong way to make a compress. Here's what you need to know:

- **Try eggs.** For eyes that have become swollen from over-exposure to the sun, beat an egg white lightly, dip a piece of gauze or sterile cotton into the liquid, and apply directly to the eyes.
- **Make a decoction.** When preparing an herbal compress, always use a decoction, not an infusion. Boiling the herb will kill microbes, which can irritate the eyes.
- **Use a filter.** Filter your decoctions carefully (two or three times) through a fine cloth to remove any filaments, twigs, dust, etc.
- **Remove your lenses.** Persons who wear contact lenses should obviously remove them before applying compresses.

Celandine is effective for improving vision. It soothes tired eyes and is recommended for the treatment of cataracts, spots on the cornea, and even retinal hemorrhaging and secretions. Simply break a stem and press the fresh sap into the corner of the eye. You can also apply fresh juice to the eyelids: Put the plant through an extractor or blender.

Lemon makes eyes shine; mix a little juice in some water and put a drop in each eye. Lemon also helps tighten loose skin under the eyes.

Eyebright decongests the eyes and combats irritation of the eyelids, tearing, and conjunctivitis. Use decoctions to prepare compresses: Boil a pinch of eyebright in a pint of water for 10 minutes. For tired swollen eyes, prepare a concentrated decoction and apply as compresses: Boil a pinch in a cup of water, then freeze into cubes; apply to the eyes and hold in place with a strip of gauze. For tearing, dab some decoction in the eyes. You can also combine eyebright with 1/3 oz each of Valerian, lilac flowers, and rue; 1/2 oz of yarrow and 1/2 oz of chamomile; mix well and soak in half a quart of cold water overnight; in the morning, heat (do not boil) and let stand for five minutes; dip sterile compresses in the decoction and leave in place for at least half an hour, adding more decoction from time to time.

Walnut helps soothe irritation and inflammation of the eyelids. Boil 2 oz of fresh leaves in a quart of water for five to seven minutes, and apply as compresses.

Onion can be combined with burdock to help alleviate swollen eyes. Prepare onion compresses using a decoction: four to six onions per quart of water.

Apple can be used to treat tired swollen eyes. Grate a raw apple, spread the pulp on a piece of gauze and apply directly to the eyes.

Potatoes help eliminate pockets under the eyes. Apply compresses a number of times a day. Grate a raw potato and apply the pulp directly to the eyes; leave in place for about 15 minutes.

Rose helps soothe red runny eyes. Apply compresses before going to bed at night. Mix equal parts of preboiled lukewarm water with rose water and soak compresses in the solution; leave in place for 15 minutes.

Rue improves vision. Use a glass container to mix a teaspoon of rue flowers with half a teaspoon of white wine and 2 oz of spring water; cover

TREATING CONJUNCTIVITIS

Ever wake up with one or both eyelids stuck together, the whites of your eyes completely bloodshot, a burning sensation, and the feeling that a foreign particle is stuck under your eyelid? If you have, then you've probably had conjuctivitis.

If these symptoms arise, always consult a doctor. While waiting for medical attention, keep your hands and toilet articles as clean as possible; avoid rubbing your eyes, no matter how much they itch; and use one of these plant remedies.

Chamomile is great for compresses that combat eye inflammation. Prepare decoctions by boiling 1/2 oz of flower tops in a liter of water for 10 minutes; filter and apply when lukewarm. You can also fill small linen bags with chamomile flowers. Heat the bags in the oven (not too hot) and apply directly to affected eyes.

Walnut is effective for treating a variety of skin problems. Apply fresh crushed walnut leaves directly to affected eyes.

Plantain is both a short- and a long-term remedy. To prepare infusions, add 2 oz of leaves to a half quart of boiling water; remove from heat, and let stand for half an hour. Dip some sterile gauze into the infusion and apply directly to the eyes for 10 minutes. To prevent recurrences, repeat the treatment every three days for three months after the condition has cleared up.

and heat in a double boiler for two hours (low heat); filter through a fine cloth and pour into a sterile container; use the mixture to bathe the eyes for three days, then prepare a new batch. Expect to wait a few weeks for results.

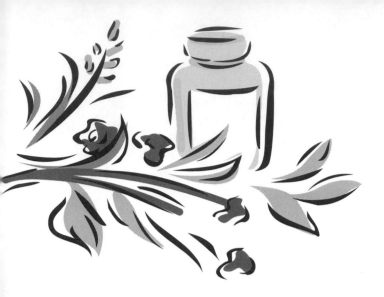

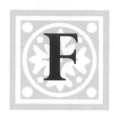

≈ Fainting

When someone faints in a crowd, it can be a frightening experience for all concerned. Unconsciousness and collapse come on suddenly, breathing all but stops, and the pulse can become so faint that it's undetectable.

Still, fainting spells don't necessarily arrive unannounced. They're often preceded by a condition known aslipothymia, characterized by feelings of general weakness and discomfort, headaches, nausea, dizziness, and ringing in the ears.

As frightening as a fainting episode may be, it doesn't necessarily point to a serious underlying cause.

FIRST AID FOR THE FAINT

In case of fainting, first aid should be administered rapidly. Don't wait for a doctor to arrive on the scene before doing anything. Loosen all tight clothing, make sure the person is getting enough air, place him or her in a prone position with the head lower than the rest of the body, and administer light slaps to the cheeks with a wet towel or cloth. You can also rub their body with warm alcohol. Next, wrap the person in a blanket or warm jacket and place a hot water bottle under their feet, if possible.

Inhalations of vinegar or smelling salts can revive someone who has fainted. Above all, don't panic, and persevere in your treatment.

People faint for many reasons: heat, general weakness, cardiac problems, intestinal parasites, and intoxication, among others. However, if you do faint, it's important to get a diagnosis from a health care professional, just to be on the safe side.

Plant Power

For fainting, there's one herbal remedy that really stands out:

Lemon balm (also called melissa) is a tonic that alleviates palpitations, anxiety, and dizziness, and inhaling lemon balm vapor can help in cases of fainting. Soak the following ingredients in a quart of water for two weeks: 3 oz of lemon balm leaves, and 1/2 oz each of lemon, dried angelica root, nutmeg powder, and coriander seeds. Add a little cinnamon and a few cloves; filter, press, and store in a sealed container. Administer one or two teaspoons at the first sign of a fainting spell.

ꙮ Fever

Remember, when you were a child, your mother's first reaction if you told her you weren't feeling well? You may have had a tummy ache, or maybe your back was hurting. It didn't matter. The response of every mother throughout the mists of time has always been the same: She put her hand on your forehead, testing for a fever.

Of course, a fever in itself isn't a problem as long as body temperature does not rise above 101.5 degrees Fahrenheit. In fact, being slightly feverish can be beneficial in many instances, as it helps eliminate toxins.

DEGREES OF FEVER

How you treat a fever depends on how high the fever is. Here are some short, simple guidelines on choosing appropriate care.

- Very mild: 98.6 to 100 degrees Fahrenheit. You can usually handle this at home.
- Mild: 100 to 101.5 degrees Fahrenheit. You can probably handle the situation at home, but check in with your doctor.
- High: 101.5 to 104 degrees Fahrenheit. A high fever can be a sign of serious infection. See a doctor as soon as possible.
- Hyperthermia: more than 104 degrees Fahrenheit. This is an emergency, possibly a life-threatening situation. Immediate professional care is a must.

KEEPING TRACK OF TEMPERATURE

Use an anal or oral thermometer to take regular readings in order to follow a fever's evolution. Reading should be taken in the morning after waking up, around noon, and in the evening at about six o'clock. Keep precise notes of the readings in case a doctor has to be called in—they will be very useful for diagnosing the type of fever and its underlying cause.

It's the underlying cause of the fever you need to be concerned about. The usual cause is an infection, but the seriousness of the infection should be determined by a health care professional. So any time you see your temperature rise by more than a degree or so, especially if you've been sick for more than a day or two, call your doctor.

Nutrition

Animals instinctively refuse to eat when they are sick. Human organisms also combat disease more effectively when nutrition is reduced to a minimum. Fasting or adopting a liquid diet composed of vegetable or fruit juice and water is an excellent idea while running a fever.

General Care

Persons with fever should stay in bed and drink a lot of liquids (pure water, lemon or grape juice). This helps lower body temperature and keep the mouth and lips moist.

Give feverish persons sponge baths and a good dry rub afterward to refresh the body and stimulate circulation. For cases of very high fever, use tepid water to help lower body temperature.

Because developing a fever always puts a strain on the body, it's always best to set some time for rest and convalescence, even after your temperature has returned to normal.

Plant Power

Plants can be highly effective for treating a fever. They help the body expel toxins and maintain strength, even with a raised temperature. Here are some to try.

Yarrow is an astringent that helps reduce fever. Use 1 oz per quart of boiling water to prepare infusions.

Angelica is a tonic and expectorant, and makes an excellent remedy for fever, because it stimulates perspiration and facilitates digestion. It is also helpful during periods of convalescence. Use 1/2 oz per quart of boiling water to prepare infusions.

Chamomile is an analgesic and tonic that helps lower fever, combats migraines and other aches and pains, and regulates stomach functions. Use 1 oz of flowers per quart of water to prepare infusions.

Centaury is known to reduce fever. It also has a depurative and antiseptic effect. Drink a cup when fever reaches its peak, and two or three cups a day after that (but only for a limited time, because the plant tends to irritate the digestive tract). Use 1/3 oz per quart of water for infusions.

Eucalyptus is a powerful antiseptic that helps decongest respiratory passages. Boil 1 oz of leaves in a quart of water for three minutes, then remove from heat and let stand for 10 minutes. Drink two or three cups a day.

Ash is a diuretic. The bark also helps reduce fever. Boil 1 to 2 oz in a quart of water for five minutes, then remove from heat and let stand for 10 minutes. Drink three cups a day, before meals.

Gentian is an aperitif that has traditionally been used to reduce intermittent fevers. One advantage to using this plant is that it's well tolerated by even the most sensitive of stomachs. Pour a quart of boiling water over 1/2 oz of ground roots; discard the water, and soak the roots in a quart of cold water for four hours. Drink a cup before or after meals (sweetened with honey if necessary).

Horehound is an expectorant that helps improve overall health and reduce fever, especially when it's intermittent. This plant can cut your recovery time in half. To alleviate bronchitis and reduce fever, drink two or three cups of infusion a day, using 1/3 oz per quart of boiling water. You can also take a pinch in powdered form, along with your meals, as the plant's active ingredients do not dissolve well in water. Horehound can be combined with angelica: 1/2 oz of horehound flower tops and 1/2 oz of angelica roots per quart of boiling water; remove from heat and let stand for 15 minutes.

Buckbean (also called bogbean) is a tonic that stimulates bodily secretions and helps reduce fever. It's recommended for cases of temporary fever associated with fatigue. Soak 3 oz of leaves in 1 1/2 quarts of water overnight, and drink three cups a day.

DEPURATIVE REMEDY FOR A FEVER

Use 1/3 oz of each of the following ingredients: powdered aloe vera, angelica root, round turmeric, rhubarb root, Chinese camphor, senna leaves, and saffron. Also use a pinch of myrrh and milk thistle. Mix all these ingredients together in a large glass container and cover with 1 1/2 quarts of good quality, 40-proof fruit alcohol. Place the container in direct sunlight or near some other heat source for 15 days. Make sure to shake or stir the mixture at least once a day. Store in your refrigerator, in a tightly sealed container.

Note: If you use this remedy to make compresses, certain precautions should be taken: (1) spread some lard, marigold ointment or petroleum jelly over the affected area; (2) use only a few drops of the depurative remedy to soak cotton compresses; (3) leave in place for two to four hours; (4) powder the affected area with talc after removing the compresses.

Orange is recommended for treating fever accompanied by insomnia, nervous spasms, stomach cramps, and coughing. It also stimulates perspiration and urination. You can use either the flowers or leaves. Boil five or six leaves in a cup of water for 10 minutes, or add a teaspoon of flowers to a cup of boiling water and infuse for 10 minutes. Drink three cups a day.

Parsley is easy to ingest and is commonly used as a condiment on all types of food. When taken as a decoction, it acts as a depurative and diuretic, and helps eliminate intestinal gas. It also combats general fatigue and urinary problems. Boil some roots in water for five minutes (seeds for three minutes), remove from heat and let stand for a few minutes. Or prepare infusions using 1 teaspoon of leaves per cup of boiling water.

Chinchona, used to make quinine, is one of the best remedies for the flu because it reduces fever and strengthens the body. Soak 1/3 oz in a quart of water for a few hours and drink two or three cups a day.

Rosemary is recommended for cases of fever accompanied by the flu. Use 2 oz per quart of water for infusions.

Sage is used in most countries around the world to combat fever. It promotes perspiration and lowers body temperature. Sage infusions also improve a patient's morale, especially if you add a pinch of ginseng, which acts as a general tonic.

A tablespoon a day of depurative remedy (see box on page 114) will help lower body temperature. The mixture is also called the Swedish Elixir, and can be used both internally and externally to treat a wide variety of disorders. Preparing infusions may seem complicated to those unfamiliar with plant remedies, but it's well worth the effort. Because the remedy is so effective, you should always keep some handy in case of emergency.

❧ Finger Infections

Like a toothache, finger infections (the medical term is *panaris*) can cause pain that seems way out of proportion to the size of the body part affected. They usually arise because of a splinter, insect bite, or some type of lesion. Many of these infections can be treated at home, but if they get deep into the skin or into the joints of the finger, a doctor's care may be necessary.

Plant Power

The first rule of care is to immerse the affected finger in water at about 100 degrees Fahrenheit two or three times a day. And remember to keep the finger well protected, especially in cold weather. Then, try these herbal remedies to get you through the rough spots.

Garlic is a powerful antiseptic. Boil some chopped or crushed cloves in milk for a few minutes, then cool and soak affected fingers in the liquid for half an hour.

Mullein softens tissues and accelerates healing. Cook leaves in milk to prepare poultices that you can apply directly to the affected finger three times a day (morning, noon, and night). Use 2 oz of plant per quart of milk; filter carefully and apply the leaves as a poultice. You can also drink the milk, which has a depurative effect.

Chamomile has a sedative, soothing effect when used internally. External applications combat inflammation: Boil 1 oz of dried leaves in a quart of water for 5 to 10 minutes; cool and bathe your fingers in the decoction a few times a day. You can also apply the leaves directly to affected fingers, held in place with some sterile gauze. When the abscess has opened, bathe the fingers in a chamomile decoction again, and then spread some St. John's wort oil (see below) on the affected area.

Marshmallow is an emollient—that is, it softens tissues and soothes inflammation and also reduces swelling. Use marshmallow compresses to accelerate the opening of abscesses. Boil 1 oz to 2 oz of roots, leaves, or flowers in a quart of water for 10 to 15 minutes; remove from heat and infuse for half an hour; apply compresses directly to affected areas.

Lavender helps alleviate pain and inflammation, and as an antiseptic combats infection. Use decoctions or lavender oil. To prepare decoctions boil 1/2 oz to 1 oz of flowers in a quart of water for 10 minutes. To make lavender oil: Soak a handful of flowers in a quart of olive oil for a couple of days (in direct sunlight or near some other heat source); filter and repeat until the oil takes on the characteristic lavender odor.

St. John's wort oil disinfects lesions and accelerates healing. Soak 1 lb of flowers in a quart of olive oil and half a quart of white wine for four days, then boil until the wine evaporates. Filter and store in a sealed container. Apply as needed.

Onion is an antiseptic that accelerates healing. Use the fine skin that separates layers of the bulb as bandages. You can also heat onion halves over hot coals or in the oven, and apply directly to affected fingers.

Horsetail is good for making a poultice: Simply crush the plant and apply, using gauze to hold in place.

☙ Fissures

Skin fissures, caused by exposure to cold, chemicals, or household products, should be treated, although they're not usually dangerous. Wearing rubber gloves is always a good idea when handling abrasive or acidic products like strong soap or even hot water.

Plant Power

Aloe vera is an excellent treatment for fissures and other types of skin problems. You can buy pure aloe vera gel in most health food stores. Apply directly to affected areas.

Oat flakes can be ground up and mixed with a little water to make a paste that softens and heals fissured skin.

Chamomile decoctions, applied externally, are another excellent treatment for skin fissures. Boil 1 oz in a quart of water for 10 minutes.

Leek juice can be mixed with a bit of hand cream and applied locally to treat fissures.

⇜ Flatulence

Flatulence. It's annoying and it's embarrassing. So how do we stop it?

The first thing to know is that it's not caused solely by what you eat.

Drinking or swallowing air while you eat, or mixing sugars and starchy foods (resulting in fermentation) will produce excessive gas. Other causes include various digestive problems, ulcers, allergies, nervous constipation, and the overuse of laxatives.

Plant Power

Fortunately, flatulence is not something you have to put up with. There are many herbal tea remedies that can do wonders when it comes to reducing gas. Here are a few to try.

Dill alleviates symptoms of aerophagia (abnormal spasmodic swallowing of air) and intestinal spasms and stimulates sluggish digestion. Drink a cup of decoction (1/3 oz of seeds per quart of water) after meals. For infants, add a teaspoon to bottles of formula.

Green aniseed is a stimulant that facilitates digestion and the passing of gas. It also alleviates painful intestinal spasms. Drinking a cup of decoction after meals helps digestion and lessens flatulence. Boil 1/2 oz of seeds in a quart of water for two minutes, and let stand for 10 minutes.

Chamomile is helpful for children suffering from gas pains. In some cases all you have to do is rub the child's stomach with a chamomile extract: Boil 2 oz of flowers in a quart of water for 20 minutes.

Cardamom stimulates sluggish digestion and circulation, soothes colic, and reduces flatulence, especially when accompanied by a sensation of cold. Eating a few cardamom seeds after a garlic-rich meal also neutralizes any unpleasant mouth odor or aftertaste. To prepare infusions, add 1 oz to a quart of boiling water; remove from heat and let stand for a few minutes.

Carrot seeds help expel gas. Infuse a pinch of seeds in a cup of water.

Caraway is an antispasmodic and anti-gas remedy that is especially recommended after overeating, as well as for cases of colic. It also stimulates the digestive system. To prepare infusions, add 2/3 oz of seeds to a quart of boiling water. Drink three cups a day.

Celery is a diuretic that stimulates kidney functions and improves muscle tone in digestive passages. Drink three cups of fresh celery juice, prepared in a juice extractor, a day. (*Note: Pregnant women should not use this remedy*).

Coriander is a stimulant that facilitates digestion and helps stop intestinal gas from building to excess. Boil one teaspoon of seeds in 12 oz of water for a couple of minutes, then remove from heat and infuse for 10 minutes.

Cumin relieves difficult, painful, or sluggish digestion, helps eliminate intestinal gas, and soothes intestinal spasms. Drink a cup of infusion after meals: 1 teaspoon of seeds per cup of boiling water; let stand for 10 minutes.

Fennel is a stimulant and anti-gas remedy that helps digestion and combats constipation. It also acts as a diuretic, and stimulates blood circulation. Drink a cup of decoction after meals. Boil 1 oz of roots in a quart of water for 10 minutes.

Lemon balm (melissa) has a calming effect, alleviating stomach cramps and difficult digestion, as well as headaches that sometimes accompany difficult digestion. It also stimulates bile secretions. Drink several cups of infusion a day, preferably after meals. Use 1 oz to 2 oz of flower tops per quart of boiling water, remove from heat and let stand for 10 minutes.

Mint is a anti-gas remedy and antispasmodic, especially for the large intestine, and helps calm digestive problems like difficult digestion, colic, and diarrhea. Drink mint tea before or after meals.

Parsley is an excellent diuretic, anti-gas remedy, antispasmodic, and depurative. It tones the digestive system and stimulates sluggish digestion. Prepare infusions using seeds if possible—1 pinch per quart of water. (*Note: Pregnant women should avoid consuming too much parsley.*)

Savory has a tonic effect. When used as a seasoning during cooking, beans and other vegetables become easier to digest, resulting in less flatulence.

Taken as an infusion, savory helps alleviate cramps and stimulates sluggish digestion. Use 2 oz per quart of water to prepare infusions, and drink a cup after meals.

Sage is a tonic for the digestive system, especially for the liver and stomach. It also helps alleviate pain and nausea. Use 2/3 oz per quart of water to prepare infusions, and drink a cup after meals.

Thyme is a stimulant, diuretic, and anti-gas remedy. It tones and stimulates sluggish digestive passages and alleviates constipation that can cause intestinal fermentation. It also has a calming effect, alleviating nervous contractions and colic, and purifies the blood. Drink about three cups of infusion a day, using 1 oz of thyme per quart of boiling water.

Wild thyme has more or less the same properties as thyme. Drink three cups a day, using 2/3 oz per quart of water to prepare infusions.

IS IT A COLD OR IS IT THE FLU?

Although their symptoms are sometimes similar, a cold and the flu are by no means the same disease. A cold will last from 7 to 10 days and disappear without a trace. The flu, on the other hand, can become a life-threatening illness. Can you tell the difference between them? Here are the symptoms:

Cold:
- Sneezing
- Coughing
- Mild fever
- Runny nose
- Sore throat and ears
- Mild chest congestion
- General feeling of fatigue and malaise

Flu:
- Muscle aches
- Fever
- Headache
- Sore throat
- Coughing with chest congestion
- Abdominal discomfort (sometimes)
- Nausea, vomiting, and diarrhea (sometimes)

Flu

The flu, or influenza as it used to be called, is very different from—and more serious than—a common cold. After an incubation period of one to three days, initial symptoms begin to appear: fatigue, aches and pains, headaches, fever between 100 and 102 degrees Fahrenheit, shivering, perspiration, and so on. The flu can cause various complications in infants and the elderly, notably sinusitis, otitis, encephalitis, or pneumonia. As we learn every year during flu season, these complications can become life threatening.

When we come down with the flu, we have to depend on our body's natural defenses to eliminate the virus. But it is a weak immune system that makes you vulnerable to the flu in the first place. Relying on analgesics like aspirin may alleviate symptoms temporarily, but that does not cure the problem. Other medications promising fast relief neither help eliminate toxins nor rebuild the immune system.

Obviously, getting a yearly flu vaccine helps. But vaccines don't always help, and sometimes we just don't get vaccinated in time.

So, then, once we're sick, how do we defend ourselves?

Nutrition

To begin with, change your eating habits.

Don't eat solid food as long as fever persists. Drink lots of orange or grapefruit juice. If your liver is affected, drink carrot juice. When fever subsides, start eating light meals, composed mainly of fruit and vegetables. Brewer's yeast, which is very rich in vitamins, is recommended as a supplement.

Plant Power

To avoid the risk of contaminating others, it's best to stay in bed. Keep warm to promote perspiration and wrap some cold compresses around your calves. Use thyme infusions to sponge your entire body once or twice a day. Then try some of these teas:

Mullein is an emollient (i.e., it reduces inflammation) that calms irritation of the mucous membranes and helps decongest breathing passages. Use about 1/2 oz of flowers per quart of water to prepare infusions; filter through some fine cheesecloth to remove filaments, which can irritate the throat; sweeten with a little honey; and drink two or three cups a day.

Cinnamon is a tonic that alleviates fatigue, especially when running a high fever. Infuse about 2 grams of bark in a cup of water for 10 minutes; drink two or three cups a day.

Couchgrass (also called doggrass) is a diuretic and a stimulant that helps kidney functions. Boil 1 oz of the plant in a little water for 10 minutes; discard the water (which is very bitter), crush the softened plant, add 1 1/4 quarts of water and boil again until only one quart remains. Add 1/3 oz of licorice and drink three cups a day.

Lemon offers excellent protection during a flu epidemic. Simply cut a lemon in half with a knife that has been sterilized in boiling water (to prevent the spread of bacteria) and squeeze into a glass of distilled water. Drink as much as you like during the course of the day.

Fennel is an aperitif and diuretic that helps combat fatigue. Drink a cup of infusion after meals: 1 oz of seeds per quart of boiling water.

Lavender is an antiseptic and diuretic. It also has a soothing effect on the stomach. Prepare decoctions using 1 oz of flowers per quart of water and drink three or four cups a day.

Rosemary is a tonic and stimulant that helps strengthen persons weakened by a flu virus. It also acts as an antiseptic and diuretic, promotes perspiration, alleviates aches and pains, and is especially beneficial for the liver. Use 1 oz to 2 oz per quart of water to prepare infusions and drink between three and five cups a day.

Goldenrod is a fast-acting diuretic that helps the body eliminate toxins and other pathogenic substances. Drink one or two cups of infusion a day.

Marigold has an antiseptic and anti-inflammatory effect. It helps eliminate toxins by stimulating perspiration. Infuse 1 oz in a quart of boiled water for 10 minutes, and drink three cups a day.

Thyme is a tonic and antiseptic that helps decongest respiratory passages, combat fatigue, and stimulate digestion. Drink five or six cups of this very pleasant-tasting infusion a day: 1/2 oz per quart of water.

Linden stimulates perspiration, and has a mildly sedative effect on the nervous system. Drink two or three cups of infusion a day.

A DELICATE BALANCE

Women should be aware that wearing high heels alters the way the body is balanced. Weight shifts dramatically forward, creating pressures on the feet that often result in deformed toes, corns, calluses, bunions, and so on. Badly fitted shoes can also result in hip deformation, spinal problems, and even gynecological difficulties. If you like wearing high heels, keep them under two inches high, except for special occasions.

Foot Problems

Each of your feet comprises 26 bones, 19 muscles, and 107 ligaments. Leonardo da Vinci called the foot "a work of art and masterpiece of engineering." Yet for all their elegance and beauty of design, we tend to ignore our feet until something goes wrong with them and they demand attention—usually with a vengeance.

Foot problems make any kind of movement extremely difficult, and can affect the rest of the body. Being unable to walk properly, for example, can cause insomnia or nervous fatigue, which in turn may lead to more serious health problems.

So the least we can do for our feet, and ourselves, is to protect them with properly fitting shoes and clean, dry socks or stockings, and to avoid putting them through the stress of wearing high heels or playing sports without the right foot gear.

Plant Power

Cashew makes a wonderful foot bath that reduces swelling: Boil 1 oz of bark in two quarts of water for 15 minutes. Wait for the brew to cool a little, then sink your feet into it, close your eyes, and enjoy!

Alder makes a soothing foot bath that relaxes feet after long hikes or spending long periods of time standing up at work. Add a handful of fresh leaves to two quarts of boiling water, remove from heat and infuse for 10 minutes.

Laurel helps alleviate the foot fatigue that you feel at the end of the day. Boil 1/2 oz of crushed berries in a quart of water, and add the decoction to your footbath. Soak your feet for 15 minutes, then dry and powder with talc.

Walnut tones and relaxes tired feet, especially during hot weather and after long walks. It also helps alleviate foot perspiration problems. Boil 1 1/2

CORNS

Although corns on your feet can be very annoying, you don't have to see a doctor to get rid of them. Even better, of course, is to keep from getting them in the first place.

To prevent corns, give your feet a chance to breathe and wear shoes that don't rub (sandals are best in summer). If you already have corns, wearing tight shoes will only make things worse.

In the treatment of corns, plants can help. Although an herbal remedy won't get rid of a corn, what it can do is soften your skin so that you can rub the corn away with a pumice stone.

Applying **garlic** directly to the skin can sometimes help. Use a bandage to keep some freshly crushed garlic on the corn overnight. Repeat the applications for 15 days.

Using **celandine** is also effective for helping to remove corns. Use the juice for regular applications, but make sure not to spread the liquid on adjoining areas of skin, because it is extremely corrosive.

oz of leaves in two quarts of water for 10 minutes (you can also add 2 oz of dried thyme); cool and soak your feet for 20 minutes. For excessive perspiration, boil 2 oz of leaves (along with 2 oz of dried thyme if you like) in a quart of water for 15 minutes. Soak your feet for at least 15 minutes, and powder with talc after drying.

Sweet flag is useful in treating chapped hands and feet, as well as cold extremities. Soak two handfuls of plant in two quarts of water overnight; bring to a boil, then cool slightly and soak affected areas for 20 minutes. For cold extremities, soak cold hands in the decoction, with the temperature as high as possible (the same decoction can be used a number of times).

Marigold can be used to treat dermatitis, fungal infections, corns, and warts. For fungal infections apply marigold ointment: Boil 3 oz of petals in 300 grams of water for 45 minutes; filter and add twice the weight of lard; simmer over low heat until the liquid has evaporated. For corns and warts, boil petals until they form a thick paste, and apply directly to affected areas (to prevent corns don't wear tight-fitting shoes).

Coltsfoot baths help reduce swelling: Add 3 oz to a quart of cold water and bring to a boil for 10 minutes.

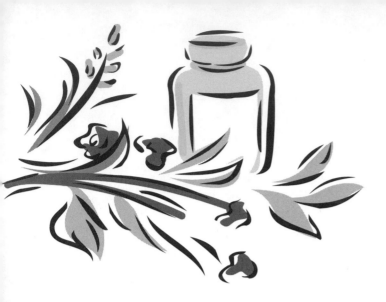

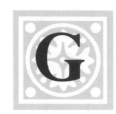

~ Gallstones

Gallstones are small stone-like objects, made of cholesterol and calcium, that grow in the liver and gallbladder. More women than men develop gallstones, so estrogen may play a role in their formation. Other causes include chronic overeating, a sedentary lifestyle, and pregnancy.

Gallstones can take a very long time to form—months or even years in some cases—and if they get too big or grow in the wrong place, they can cause problems. These include difficult digestion, frequent nausea and bloating, and pain on the right side of the stomach. At the extreme, high temperature and an increased white blood cell count could indicate an inflammation of the gallbladder that requires surgical treatment.

Intense pain can become overwhelming if the stone starts to move down the bile duct, which is a long tube that carries a digestive chemical called bile that's manufactured by the gallbladder. With the duct blocked, the gallbladder cannot empty itself, and it becomes swollen with its own secretions.

In any case, if you suspect you have a gallstone, be sure to see a doctor.

Nutrition

Because the gallbladder and liver are both parts of the digestive system, what foods you eat and how you eat them will obviously have a great effect on the health of these organs. To avoid forming gallstones, try following these tips.

Chew your food thoroughly. Food that is mixed with saliva and chewed to a pulp before being swallowed is much easier to digest.

Reduce your salt intake. Don't use table salt, and avoid foods that contain hidden salts, such as processed meats; salted, marinated, or smoked meat or fish; heavy sauces; canned goods; etc. Also avoid pork, pressed meat and sausages, white flour and sugar, spicy foods, brussels sprouts, asparagus, spinach, and rhubarb.

Drink lots of spring water. Good, clean water will help to flush out and detoxify your system.

WHAT TO DO IN CASE OF A GALLBLADDER ATTACK

Pain from a gallstone can be extreme. Get the person to take a hot bath for about half an hour. After the bath keep the person warm with infusions of chicory (or another of the herbs listed on page 126). Then take another half-hour bath, and so on. Try using massage to gently help the stone move along. Pain will subside as the stone gets close to the end of its journey—the urinary bladder. If the person has a heart condition, place cold compresses on his or her forehead and wrists.

When the attack subsides, administer sitz baths to make sure the stone does not stay in the bladder, where it can cause irritation and bleeding. If the stone is not passed naturally, surgery is the only option. Chicory infusions can help pass a stone that has reached the bladder.

General Care

In some cases ingesting oil, which in turn stimulates abundant bile secretions, can help eliminate stones that are stuck in the urethra. This technique is effective if stones are not too large. Use unrefined olive, sunflower seed, or hazelnut oil. Start by cleaning out your stomach—swallow some freshly ground linseed or a few soaked figs, or use a chamomile decoction as an enema. For the oil treatment to be effective, you have to drink at least 10 fluid ounces at a time. After taking the oil, lie down on your right side for at least two hours. Eliminating stones in this way is much easier on the body than surgery.

Plant Power

Agrimony is an astringent and decongestant that helps eliminate gallstones when used as an extended cure (best in summer when you can obtain the fresh plant). Place 1 oz in a quart of water, cover, and boil over low heat for five minutes; remove from heat and let stand for 10 minutes. Drink four or five small cups a day.

Artichoke is recommended as a cure for gallstones and intense pain from the liver. Use 1 oz of leaves (not stems) per quart of water to prepare decoctions. Because of the very bitter taste, some people prefer artichoke tincture: Soak 1 lb of dried cut leaves in a quart of eau-de-vie or brandy for 15 days; press, filter, and store in a sealed container. Take two teaspoons before meals, mixed with a little water.

Wild chicory is a diuretic and intestinal antiseptic that stimulates bile secretions. Chicory infusions can help dissolve gallstones, even during a crisis: Use a pinch to 1/3 oz of dried leaves, or 1 oz of non-roasted dried roots per quart of water.

Couchgrass (also called doggrass) is a diuretic, depurative, and anti-inflammatory for the urinary tract. It helps alleviate both hepatic and renal colic. Boil 1 oz of couchgrass in a little water. Discard the water, crush the rhizomes, and boil them again in 1 1/4 quarts of water until a half pint has evaporated. Add zest of lemon or a teaspoon of licorice to flavor, and drink up to a quart a day. (You can also add another diuretic plant to the decoction.)

Linseed has a soothing effect on inflamed urinary passages and helps eliminate gallstones. To prepare infusions, use 2/3 oz of linseed per quart of water and drink four or five cups a day. You can also soak 2/3 oz of linseed in a quart of water overnight. Flavor with licorice or another diuretic plant.

Dandelion is a diuretic and depurative that aids in the evacuation of the bile ducts and helps eliminate gallstones. To prepare infusions, use 1 oz to 2 oz of fresh or dried leaves per quart of water. Drink three to six cups per day, for a period of one week. If you want to use the roots, prepare decoctions: Boil 2 oz of finely chopped roots in a quart of water for five minutes. You can also eat fresh stems to stimulate the liver and gallbladder, which in some cases is enough to reabsorb smaller stones. Eat dandelion salad twice a day for a period of two weeks.

Black radish is an excellent treatment for gallstones, on condition that you don't have a fragile or irritated digestive system. Sip small amounts of juice throughout the day for a period of six weeks (use a juice extractor to prepare fresh juice). Start with 3 oz of juice before breakfast, increasing the amount gradually over a three-week period, to 12 oz. Then gradually reduce the amount to 3 oz over a second three-week period. You can also take a third of a wine glass composed of half carrot juice and half black radish juice, a quarter of an hour before meals.

❧ Gangrene

The word "gangrene" conjures images of amputation and painful death, and with good reason. Tissue that is deprived of blood, and therefore of oxygen, will die. That's what happens to persons with gangrene. Affected tissue will become shiny, bluish and hard to the touch, but under no circumstances should you wait for that to happen if you suspect you may be developing gangrene. Consult a doctor immediately.

General Care

Blood circulation must be reestablished, so keep moving around as much as possible while waiting to see a doctor. Stay warm.

Plant Power

The plants listed below can be helpful in reestablishing circulation to affected tissue, but once again, using these remedies is only a stopgap measure until the doctor arrives.

Garlic helps stimulate circulation and purifies the blood. Boil two or three crushed cloves in one and a half cups of water or milk.

Wormwood is an antiseptic that helps heal gangrenous wounds. Use fresh sap, or prepare decoctions: Boil 2 oz to 3 oz of the plant in a quart of water for 10 minutes. You can also prepare a tincture: Soak a cup of dried plant in a quart of alcohol heated to 140 degrees Fahrenheit.

❧ Gout

Gout is an inflammatory joint disorder, usually of the toes, caused by an increased amount of uric acid in the blood. The problem seems to be hereditary, affecting mainly men past the age of 50 who have spent a lifetime indulging themselves with rich food and alcohol. Emotional setbacks or tension can sometimes trigger attacks.

Initial symptoms of an attack include indigestion, general fatigue, and cramps in the affected toe. Persons are often awakened in the middle of the night as pain in the big toe intensifies to the point where it becomes excruciating.

Nutrition

During attacks stick to a liquid diet: water, herbal tea, and vegetable broth. Make sure to avoid foods that contain large amounts of cholesterol, like butter, cheese, and beef.

Lifestyle

There isn't much you can do during an attack except stay in bed and take pain killers. However, once the crisis has passed, there are steps you can take to prevent—or at least postpone—recurrences. Leading a balanced, regular life and not straining yourself with too much work or worry will help prevent recurrences in chronic cases. Also try to avoid extremes of cold or humidity.

Plant Power

Along with changes in lifestyle, herbal remedies can help prevent future gout attacks from taking place. Here are some to try.

Burdock is a depurative and diuretic that helps eliminate toxins that have accumulated in the body. Use leaves to prepare infusions and roots to prepare decoctions. Drink two or three cups a day.

Birch is a powerful diuretic. Use 2 oz per quart of water to prepare infusions, and drink between three and five cups a day, with or between meals.

Celery is an excellent condiment for persons suffering from gout, because it helps prevent recurring attacks.

Ash is a diuretic and tonic that lowers uric acid levels in the blood, thus eliminating toxins and combating rheumatic problems like gout and other types of joint pain. It's also recommended for persons who are suffering from fatigue or convalescing after a prolonged illness. Use 1 oz per quart of water to prepare infusions, and drink three cups a day.

Wild pansy is another depurative that helps combat gout. Soak 1 oz in a quart of water for two hours; then bring to a boil, remove from heat, and let stand for 10 minutes. Drink three or four cups a day (reduce the dosage if the infusion has a laxative effect or makes you feel like vomiting).

Queen of the meadow has a tonic and diuretic effect, and helps eliminate accumulated toxins. Place a teaspoon of flowers (tops are best) in a cup of hot water (not more than 175 degrees Fahrenheit) and let stand for a few minutes. Make sure not to boil the flowers. Combining queen of the meadow with ash and black currant (2/3 oz of each per quart of water) makes an even more effective remedy for gout.

Fleabane reduces inflammation and helps prevent rheumatic problems. The plant is also a diuretic that aids in the elimination of uric acid. Use a tablespoon per cup of boiling water to prepare infusions. Sweeten with honey and drink three cups a day, between meals.

Depurative remedy helps cure gout. Add a teaspoon of the remedy (Appendix A) to a cup of horsetail and nettle infusion (1 oz of each per quart of water); drink three cups a day.

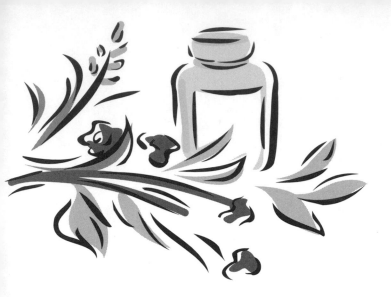

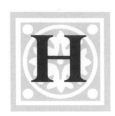

✒ Hair Problems

Let's face it. Limp, damaged, or thinning hair doesn't threaten your life, keep you bedridden, or send you running for pain killers. The only thing it hurts is your vanity. But vanity—or at least confidence and self-esteem—can be extremely important to your emotional health. So if your hair is giving you trouble, you needn't feel embarrassed about making some efforts to remedy the situation.

Nutrition

The health and beauty of your hair doesn't depend solely on the products you use to care for it. Your lifestyle and the kinds of foods you eat also have an affect. Here are the three essentials of a healthy hair diet.

Take the right vitamins. Make sure you're getting enough Vitamins A, B, and C. Vitamin B5 (pantothenic acid) is especially important, as it's reputed to prevent hair loss and discoloration.

Don't forget your minerals. Iron, iodine, and copper are three important minerals for maintaining healthy hair. Iodine is essential for thyroid functions, one of which is to ensure proper circulation, thus nourishing the scalp and preventing hair loss. Garlic and kelp (a type of algae) are very rich in iodine (*Caution: Obese persons should not absorb too much iodine*).

Desalinate. Avoid consuming too much salt, which can cause hair loss.

ESSENTIAL CARE FOR BEAUTIFUL HAIR

Keeping your hair lustrous, vibrant, and attractive is easy. It's a matter of following a few simple rules. Here's what to do.

Massage your scalp every day. It stimulates blood circulation. Start at the base of your neck and work upward, forming small circles with the tips of your fingers.

Avoid chemical hair products. These include dyes, shampoos, and bleaching agents. Opt for mild herbal shampoos, and use only a small amount: 1 or 2 teaspoons per wash. Don't forget that rinsing your hair well is just as important as washing.

Use a good hair brush. The best are made from nylon bristles, spaced well apart, with rounded tips, and set in a flexible rubber base. This kind of brush massages the scalp without damaging hair. If you use a comb, make sure the teeth are widely spaced, and don't use metal combs.

Protect your hair from extremes. Don't dry your hair with your hair dryer set too hot. Shield your scalp from direct sunlight, salt, wind, and spray by wearing scarves or hats. Use a swimming cap if you swim in chlorinated water a lot. If you swim in the ocean, wash the salt out of your hair at the end of the day.

Plant Power

Plants offer a wide range of effective products that can improve the condition of your hair. Here are just a few.

Burdock decoctions, taken internally, help keep the scalp healthy and add luster to dull-looking hair. You can also use burdock to rinse your hair after shampooing or as a scalp lotion for massages. To prepare your decoctions, boil 2 oz of chopped roots in a quart of water for 10 minutes. To prepare a scalp lotion, add 3 oz of freshly chopped burdock to half a quart of rum.

Chamomile is recommended for blond hair. The plant restores luster and gives hair a pleasant odor. To prepare a scalp lotion, soak 1 oz of dried flowers in a quart of water overnight. You can also use a concentrated chamomile decoction to rinse your hair after washing: 2 oz of flowers, boiled in a quart of water for 20 minutes, and filtered.

Onions are helpful in the treatment of almost any type of scalp problem. Rub your scalp with a fresh onion (cut in half) before shampooing. You can

NATURAL SHAMPOOS AND RINSES

In a world where commercial hair products are so numerous they nudge each other off the store shelves, it's good to know you can make a natural shampoo or rinse of your own that smells better, works better, and costs less.

The formulas are simple. Use chamomile, mullein, or nettle for blond or light brown hair; marjoram, parsley, and/or cinnamon for dark brown hair; hibiscus, juniper, or sage for red hair; lavender, sage, rosemary, or thyme for black hair. Prepare infusions or decoctions (boil for 10 minutes) using 1 oz of the plant of your choice per half quart of water. Let stand overnight, then pour into an enamel or stainless steel container and add 1 oz of grated castile soap (this type of soap will not remove your hair's natural oils). Heat while stirring constantly; then remove from heat and cool to a lukewarm temperature, adding one or two drops of essential oil of the plant recommended for your hair type. Store in a warm location, because the mixture will solidify in the cold.

To get an all natural rinse, first use cider vinegar after shampooing to rinse out all the soap. Then rinse again with thyme, sage, or rosemary to tone your scalp (thyme is especially effective). Use a decoction: Boil 1 oz of the plant in a quart of water over low heat for 20 minutes. For a final rinse, use lemon mixed with water to make your hair more supple and lustrous.

also rub some lanolin into your scalp. If you find the odor too strong, buy a commercial onion lotion at your local pharmacy or health food store.

Nettle is beneficial for treating all types of hair problems. Massaging regularly with nettle tincture improves the vitality of your hair, gets rid of dandruff, and helps prevent hair loss. To prepare a scalp lotion, use 3 oz of a mixture of nasturtium leaves and seeds, fresh nettle leaves, and fresh boxtree; chop the leaves and soak in half a quart of 90-proof alcohol for 15 days; filter (through a press if possible) and mix the juice thus obtained with a quart of spring water. Rub into the scalp morning and night.

Leek infusions do the same thing for brown and reddish hair that chamomile does for blond hair. Use a pinch of seeds infused in a cup of boiled water for 10 minutes.

Sage infusions stimulate hair growth. Applied as a lotion, the plant nourishes the scalp and prevents hair loss. Rinse with infusions: 1 oz of dried

SPECIAL HAIR PROBLEMS

A few of us are lucky enough to have hair that is neither too oily nor too dry—a very few of us. The rest of us have to cope with whatever kind of bad hair day our particular scalps have on the menu. But we're not helpless. Here are some suggestions for turning unruly tangles into elegant tresses.

Dry Hair

Prepare a shampoo (see page 132) using burdock, sage, or quince seeds. Then add two egg yolks and one teaspoon of almond oil, mixed in a blender. Shampoo twice, then rinse with the appropriate plant. Between shampoos, rub a few drops of essential oil of chamomile (for light hair) or rosemary (for dark hair) on your hands, then coat your hair brush with the oil and brush your hair, from the roots outward. Also protect your hair against direct sunlight.

Greasy Hair

Prepare the castile soap shampoo (see page 132), using lavender, mint, marigold, or yarrow. Don't use too much shampoo, and rinse with a plant-based decoction that is right for your hair color, adding a teaspoon of cider vinegar to the mixture.

Dull, Brittle Hair

Boil 2/3 oz of sage in a quart of water for 20 minutes. Filter and press well, then add the juice of half a lemon. Use the preparation as a final rinse.

sage in a quart of boiled water, infused for 15 minutes. To prepare a scalp lotion, use equal parts of sage tincture (available in herbal and health food stores) and rum. Rub into the scalp daily.

✎ Hay Fever

Ah, the sights and sounds of crisp October: watery eyes, runny noses, and the ubiquitous "Achoo!" Ragweed is blooming, and the air is full of mold spores. It's hay fever time.

Of course, hay fever can also occur in the spring when there's lots of pollen in the air. And in the summer, when there's plenty of dust. Staying indoors won't help you either, if you happen to have pets and you're sensitive to their dander.

So what do you do?

General Care

Curing hay fever is a complex matter, because it has so many causes, and the immune system—which gives you your symptoms—is itself extremely complicated. But there are some steps you can take.

Do it by hand. For immediate relief, press on the following acupuncture points with your fingertips: the middle of the forehead, behind the hairline, and under the nostrils.

Clear the air. A negative ion device installed in your home and/or workplace can be very helpful in taking allergens out of the air.

Build resistance. Once an allergen has been identified, people can take very small amounts of the same substance in order to build up an immunity. This should be done under a doctor's care only. It usually takes several months before results become apparent.

Plant Power

Herbal remedies can be quite helpful in relieving the discomfort of hay fever. Here are the best ones to try.

Goldenseal combats inflammation and has a beneficial effect on mucous membranes lining the respiratory passages. To treat inflammation, sniff some powdered goldenseal leaves. To prepare decoctions, boil 1 oz of flower tops in a quart of milk, then remove from heat and let stand for 15 minutes; sweeten with honey and drink two or three cups a day.

Ground ivy soothes irritation of mucous membranes and stimulates expectoration. Infuse 1 oz of dried plant in a quart of water for 10 minutes, and drink three or four cups a day.

Goldenrod is an effective treatment for allergies. Pour a quart of boiling water over 2 oz of flower tops, boil for 10 minutes, then remove from heat and let stand for 12 hours; filter and drink half a quart a day.

Headaches

Although most headaches are benign, you shouldn't ignore them. Simple tension or eye strain can cause them, but so can high or low blood pressure, infections, and brain diseases.

Plant Power

For garden variety headaches—ones that come from tension or being overtired—try these remedies from the garden.

Windflower is a sedative and antispasmodic that should be used prudently, because it's toxic in large doses. Soak a handful of the plant in an equal amount of 95-proof alcohol for eight days; store in a cool location and agitate from time to time; press, filter, and take 20 to 40 drops a day.

Rumanian chamomile is a tonic, antispasmodic, and pain killer. Take it in powdered form (a pinch every four hours) or prepare infusions using 1 oz per quart of water; drink a cup (unsweetened) a half hour before meals.

German chamomile has much the same properties as

WHAT KIND OF HEADACHE IS IT?

Most headaches can be classified into one of three types: tension, migraine, or cluster.

Tension headaches occur when the muscles of your neck or scalp contract. It can result from stress, depression, anything that makes you hold your head in one position for a long time—like reading or using a computer or even sleeping in a cold room.

Migraine headaches are more severe. They can be preceded by visual disturbances like flashing lights; waving, scintillating lines; or blind spots. The headache itself is usually throbbing, and most often occurs on one side of the head. Dizziness, nausea, vomiting, and extreme fatigue are also common. Migraines will usually last from 6 to 48 hours. They're more common in women than men, and can be related to anything from a family history of migraine to the consumption of foods you're sensitive to.

Cluster headaches are severe and come on suddenly, often during the REM (dreaming) phase of sleep. They're more common in men. No one knows what causes them, but they seem to be related to the release of a substance called histamine into the blood. They've been known to occur in some patients on a daily basis for over a year. Alcohol and tobacco have been known to trigger cluster episodes, as have sun glare and foods to which individuals have shown sensitivity.

Rumanian chamomile, but also helps regulate menstrual flow. Use 2/3 oz per quart of water to prepare infusions, and let stand for 20 minutes.

❧ Heartburn

The symptoms of heartburn are all too familiar: an uncomfortable burning sensation in your throat and chest, and sometimes belching, usually after meals. They're so familiar, in fact, that sometimes we don't take them seriously. But they can signal more than simply a meal that didn't agree with you. The symptoms may be telling you that you have a stomach ulcer, and if they become chronic, medical intervention may become necessary.

General Care

People who tend to suffer from gastric acidity, which is the basic problem underlying heartburn, should adopt a relatively tranquil lifestyle and avoid potential sources of emotional tension. However, because we are not always in a position to avoid these situations, it's a good idea to practice some form of relaxation technique like yoga. In short, try not to get involved in incessant arguments or worry too much. Calm is always best.

Lifestyle

Heartburn can be very responsive to changes in your daily habits and lifestyle. Here are some ways to make a difference in your stomach's health right now.

Avoid antacids. Although they may alleviate symptoms temporarily, they do nothing to solve the underlying problem, resulting in more frequent recurrences.

Don't smoke. Tobacco products can be hard on the tummy. Smoke as little as possible, and resolve to stop smoking altogether as soon as you can.

Take a siesta. People all over the world seem to know the advantages to napping after meals, but it's not a custom we've adopted in America. We should. It aids the digestion and refreshes us for the rest of the day.

Dress comfortably. Don't wear clothing that's too tight and tends to

YOUR STOMACH IS NO PLACE FOR ATMOSPHERE

Swallowing air, technically known as aerophagy, isn't dangerous, but it certainly can be annoying. It can even cause stomach bloating and frequent belching which, in certain situations, can be embarrassing to say the least.

The remedy, fortunately, is as easy as 1-2-3:

1. **Savor your food.** Eat slowly and chew thoroughly, in a calm environment. That will keep you from gulping down food and air together. Think about what you are doing instead of watching TV, reading a newspaper, or getting involved in discussions about business or politics.

2. **Stop smoking.** Now there's advice you never hear. But the fact is, the more you smoke, the more saliva you swallow, and the more air you swallow with it.

3. **Say goodbye to gas producers.** Stop drinking coffee and strong alcohol, and avoid stews, cabbage, radishes, soft white bread, potatoes, strong spices, and soft drinks.

inhibit circulation (tight belts, tight underwear). The better you circulate blood, the better your digestive tract operates.

Nutrition

Try to eat slowly, and chew your food thoroughly (this applies to everyone, whether you suffer from stomach problems or not). Eat healthy foods that are not too spicy, and cut down on your salt intake.

Look for foods that contain Vitamins D and B6 (sometimes called Vitamin G—consult the section on Vitamins and Minerals for more details), and eat curd, which is excellent for regulating and neutralizing stomach acids.

Drinking brown rice water is also an excellent way to reduce gastric acidity. Rinse some cooked brown rice thoroughly in a little water, then set the water aside and drink small amounts throughout the course of the day.

Acidic Offenders

Obviously, what you eat can give you heartburn. So here are some common food offenders to cut back on or avoid if you want to keep your tummy calm and feeling good:

• Processed meats

WHAT TO DO FOR SLUGGISH DIGESTION

People often feel heavy and sleepy after eating, especially after a copious meal accompanied by wine.

To prevent sluggish digestion, chew your food well and don't eat a lot of bread during meals. If you experience heartburn or stomach pain, drink alcohol only between meals instead of while eating.

Brewer's yeast is a food supplement that is excellent for your digestion. The B-complex vitamins and proteins it contains stimulate contractions of your digestive system, which in turn produces more digestive juices, facilitating the evacuation of waste.

Smokers should make every effort not to smoke before breakfast, and wait as long as possible afterward before having their first cigarette.

If you follow this advice, and if your diet is well balanced and you don't stuff yourself, you should not experience sensations of heaviness or somnolence after meals.

- Canned meat or fish
- Mayonnaise and mustard
- Hard cheeses
- White bread and other white flour products
- Spinach, celery, and radishes
- Deep-fried foods
- Fatty foods
- Alcohol
- Acidic foods such as grapefruit and rhubarb
- Vinegar
- White sugar (use natural honey to sweeten your foods instead)

Plant Power

To reduce stomach acid, one herb stands out among all others.

Sweet flag needs to be prepared cold. Soak a teaspoon in a cup of cold water overnight; in the morning, warm up the liquid slightly using a steamer, and strain; drink a mouthful before and after meals (not more than six times a day).

≫ Hemorrhoids

Hemorrhoids are actually burst blood vessels in the anus. Various factors can cause the problem: a lack of exercise; chronic constipation; rectal irritation resulting from hard, dry stool; a weak liver; or high blood pressure.

Nutrition

Adopt a hypotoxic diet. Brewer's yeast, rich in B vitamins and proteins, improves digestive functions and stimulates the secretion of digestive juices, which, in turn, facilitate the elimination of solid waste. If your problem is constipation, don't do anything drastic to remedy the situation, because you might only make matters worse. Instead, try a gradual approach that treats the underlying cause. One aspect of such an approach is to make some dietary changes: Eat more green vegetables and avoid nitrogenous greasy foods, sweets, and fermented drinks.

General Care

If bleeding occurs, you'll need to make sure that the problem is really a hemorrhoid, so see a doctor. Other, more serious disorders (polyps, dysentery, colitis, and even cancer) can present many of the same symptoms as a hemorrhoid.

If pain becomes intense, an olive oil suppository will facilitate the evacuation of stool in about half an hour (it's best to use a bedpan and eliminate stool in a prone position). After elimination, bathe the rectal region with some cotton swabs dipped in lukewarm water that has been previously boiled; then use another cotton swab to apply some olive or sweet almond oil. Two or three cold enemas a week will also be of benefit, as will an occasional sitz bath (see page 140).

Avoid remaining in a standing or sitting position for too long a time (especially on soft couches or armchairs) and exercise moderately on a regular basis.

Plant Power

Yarrow is a coagulant that will prevent hemorrhoids from bleeding profusely. It also acts as an antiseptic and will reduce bleeding over the long term. Use the freshly ground plant or an ointment (which has the advantage

SITZ BATH FOR HEMORRHOIDS

One way to relieve the pain of hemorrhoids is to take sitz baths. For best results, you should take two a day, one in the morning and one at night (lukewarm in summer, hot in winter).

- **Pain-relief formula:** To alleviate hemorrhoid pain, use a handful of witch hazel leaves mixed with 1 oz of milk thistle roots and leaves and 1 oz of lavender flowers; boil in two quarts of water for 10 minutes, filter and cool to the desired temperature.
- **Inflammation-reducing formula:** Boil 1 oz of mullein flowers, 1 oz of pellitory, and 1 oz of elder in two quarts of water for 10 minutes; filter and cool to the desired temperature.

of lasting longer) for external applications: Finely chop 2/3 oz each of fresh yarrow flowers and raspberry leaves and add to 3 oz of lard or petroleum jelly; warm over low heat until liquid, then remove from heat and let stand overnight; reheat the next day and filter through a fine cloth; store in a sealed container, and keep the ointment cool. To prepare infusions, use 2/3 oz per quart of water, and add a pinch of aniseed to neutralize the rather strong taste.

Bistort is an astringent that helps soothe hemorrhoid pain and tighten tissues. Apply compresses soaked in a bistort infusion twice a day, leaving in place for 15 minutes. Use 2 oz of roots per quart of water.

Mullein soothes irritation. Use it to prepare sitz baths and compresses: Boil 1 oz of leaves and flowers in a quart of water for five minutes.

Witch hazel, added to sitz baths (see box above), helps alleviate hemorrhoid pain.

Pellitory has a soothing, emollient effect and is recommended for hemorrhoids accompanied by anal fissures. Prepare poultices using the freshly ground plant, or compresses soaked in a concentrated infusion: 2 oz of plant per quart of water.

Horsetail has a coagulant and healing effect. Use it to prepare compresses, especially for painful clustered hemorrhoids. Grind up some fresh, washed horsetail using a mortar and pestle; apply directly to the affected area or prepare a decoction: Boil 3 oz of plant in a quart of water for 15 minutes.

～ Herpes

Herpes. Now there's a word nobody likes to hear. But the hard fact is, most of us are carrying around a herpes virus of one kind or another. About 25 percent of us have genital herpes, and a whopping 9 out of 10 of us have oral herpes. Scary.

Fortunately, herpes infections are generally benign, although they can be unpleasant and even extremely painful. And to make matters more annoying, the problem is chronic, so attacks will probably recur throughout your life.

A note of warning: There is one group of people for whom herpes can be serious and even fatal: newborns. If you are pregnant and suspect you are carrying the herpes virus, make absolutely certain that you consult a doctor.

Lifestyle

Persons carrying the herpes virus are more likely to suffer outbreaks when they are under a lot of stress or emotional pressure. The virus also tends to flare up while women are menstruating. Therefore, in addition to internal and external treatments, it might by a good idea to practice some form of relaxation or meditation.

Plant Power

Although there is no known cure for herpes, there are some things you can do to make outbreaks less frequent and less painful, and even to make herpes sores go away faster. Here are some remedies to try.

Burdock has a depurative and antiseptic effect, and can be used for both internal and external applications. Try to obtain some fresh roots, or a stabilized extract, available at health food and herbal stores. For local applications, soak a handful of leaves in olive oil. You can also boil 2 oz of burdock and 2 oz of nettle in a quart of water for an hour (adding water to compensate for evaporation); drink three small cups a day, and use the liquid to prepare compresses for local applications.

Fumitory has a depurative and calming effect. Use 2 oz of plant per quart of water to prepare infusions, and drink a cup each day before breakfast.

Malva has a calming effect and helps soothe irritation when herpes pustules are painful and inflamed. Prepare hot poultices by steaming fresh leaves or crushed roots.

≫ Hiccups

Hiccups are the result of involuntary contractions of the diaphragm. This pushes enough air up through the vocal chords to produce the characteristic hiccup sound. What causes them? Anything from alcohol consumption to eating dry, starchy foods.

What gets rid of them? Everyone has a favorite technique, from holding your breath, drinking a glass of water while bending over, to swallowing a tablespoon of pineapple juice. If any of these techniques work for you, all the better!

Plant Power

Absinthe is an antispasmodic that stops contractions of the diaphragm. It also has a beneficial effect on digestion in general. Infuse a pinch of absinthe in a quart of boiling water for five minutes, and sweeten with a little honey. Drink two cups a day, hot or cold, for a period of three days to treat persistent hiccups. *Note: Absinthe can be habit forming, so do not exceed the recommended dosage.*

Angelica is another antispasmodic plant that facilitates digestion. Use 1/2 oz of seeds per quart of water to prepare infusions.

Mint is an antispasmodic that has a calming effect on the nervous system, stimulates stomach functions, and helps prevent intestinal fermentation and the formation of excess gas. If you tend to get the hiccups after eating, drink a cup of mint infusion before leaving the table: Use 2/3 oz of plant per quart of boiling water.

✑ High Blood Pressure

High blood pressure, or hypertension, is sometimes called "the silent killer." You can have it for years and never know it, while the whole time it puts you at greater risk for heart attack, hardening of the arteries, stroke, kidney damage, and a host of other serious problems.

You can buy a device at your local pharmacy that accurately measures blood pressure. There are two numbers that must be taken into account: systolic tension, which refers to blood pressure at the moment the heart contracts; and diastolic tension, which refers to blood pressure between two heart contractions. Generally, a reading of 120/80 is considered normal, and consistent readings above 140/90 indicate hypertension.

Symptoms

We should always listen to our body. Past the age of 50, the following symptoms may indicate that you have high blood pressure: frequent

---

THE BLOOD PRESSURE DIET

There is a diet expressly designed to lower blood pressure that has proven extremely effective. The Kempner Diet, as it's called, is completely natural and highly therapeutic. Although somewhat strict, it can bring your blood pressure back to normal in just three months and eliminate symptoms like headaches, dizziness, and numbness. Here's what to do.

- Breakfast: 3 oz of rice sweetened with honey or fructose; a small glass of prune juice; a cooked apple; a grapefruit.
- 10 A.M. snack: half a glass of orange juice and a bunch of grapes.
- Lunch: rice sweetened with honey; half a glass of orange juice; a ripe banana; six slices of apple, one slice of pineapple, and a handful of raisins, dried apricots, or peaches.
- Supper: rice sweetened with honey, 2/3 cup of orange juice, four or five figs, and half an orange or some apricots.
- 9 P.M.: half a glass of orange juice.

As you can see, the diet is very low in fat (lipids) and high in slow assimilation sugars (glucides). It's also rich in protein and contains no salt (rice is steamed or boiled, without salt), canned foods, or nuts (hazelnuts, almonds, peanuts, etc.). Drink a maximum of one quart a day of liquids. After three months, you can resume a less severe hypotoxic diet.

headaches or dizziness, vision problems, ringing in the ears, insomnia, and involuntary movements of the body right after waking up. However, these symptoms are not specific to hypertension. Other things can cause them as well. So getting your blood pressure checked regularly, with or without symptoms, is important.

Nutrition

Here's what to avoid: fatty meat (beef, pork, processed meats, stews, liver paté, brains, sweetbreads), butter, cream, fermented cheeses, alcohol, coffee, tea, and wheat germ.

Replace eggs, cheese, meat, and even legumes with buckwheat or natural rice whenever possible. Garlic is known to lower blood pressure, so cook with garlic whenever possible. You can add a lot of fresh garlic to your salads, or eat steamed garlic cloves as a vegetable side-dish.

Plant Power

Although homeopathy can be an effective treatment for hypertension, especially as far as prevention is concerned, your best bet, aside from allopathic medications prescribed for very severe cases, is probably plants. The following list includes diuretics and herbs that help you relax, both of which will reduce blood pressure over the long run.

Garlic is a recommended treatment for atherosclerosis (hardening of the arteries) and all types of hypertension. Laboratory research has confirmed the popular belief that garlic does actually lower blood pressure. Use garlic drops, garlic capsules (to avoid the characteristic odor), or drink garlic infusions. Thirty drops a day for a period of 10 days a month is usually enough to lower blood pressure; soak 3 oz of garlic in half a quart of 60-proof alcohol for 10 days; stir regularly, then filter and press.

Wild garlic is also effective for lowering blood pressure. It also helps prevent the calcification of arteries, cures some types of heart problems, and has a depurative effect. Add wild garlic to salads and cooked foods especially when in season. You can also prepare a wild garlic liquor: Fill a container with fresh leaves or finely chopped cloves and cover with 40-proof alcohol; let stand in a warm place or in direct sunlight for 15 days; take 10 to 15 drops diluted in a glass of water, four times a day.

TOP 10 HEALTH HABITS FOR BEATING HYPERTENSION

1. Avoid stressful situations and overly intense physical effort.

2. Stay out of the hot sun, and remember that altitudes above 4500 feet can be harmful.

3. Practice a relaxation or meditation technique.

4. Eat a number of smaller meals instead of three large meals a day. Smaller amounts of food are easier for your body to assimilate, and place less of a strain on your digestive system.

5. Eat less butter, oil, and fat. Adopt a hypotoxic diet, if you can.

6. Eat only three meat dishes a month.

7. Make natural, whole grain rice a staple of your diet.

8. Drink 1 1/2 quarts of liquid a day, including water, tea, etc.

9. Cut down on your salt intake. You can eliminate salt from your diet completely, except for one or two days a month (to prevent a deficiency). Season foods with lemon, garlic, and sunflower seed or corn oil.

10. Use garlic. It's remarkably beneficial for treating hypertension. Use it in soups, salads, main dishes, as a spread on toast.

Hawthorn is a natural fortifier that tones and regulates the heart. It also has a tranquilizing and antispasmodic effect. Hawthorn lowers blood pressure, especially in cases of neuro-arthritic hypertension, and can also be used to treat hypotension (low blood pressure) and atherosclerosis, without producing any of the harmful side effects so common among conventional medications. Hawthorn dilates the arteries, and acts as a sedative for frayed nerves. *Note, however, that this plant should not be used for an extended period of time, because it can inhibit normal heart and liver functions.* To avoid these effects, all you have to do is stop taking the plant for a few days, say one week out of every month. Boil 2 oz of flowers and berries in a quart of water for three minutes and drink three cups a day, three weeks per month.

Mistletoe dilates the blood vessels and is an excellent heart tonic. It improves circulation and is effective for combating both hypertension and hypotension, especially when associated with problems of dizziness or irregular heartbeat. Mistletoe is also recommended for the treatment of problems related to kidney disorder, menopause, or atherosclerosis, and has a calming antispasmodic effect. Soak 1 oz in a quart of cold water overnight; heat to the boiling point (no more), and drink three cups a day, taking small sips between meals.

Maté is a Peruvian herb that acts as a diuretic and heart tonic. It helps eliminate toxins, combats fatigue, and tones the nervous system. Use 2/3 oz per quart of water to prepare infusions, and drink three cups a day.

Yarrow dilates the blood vessels and helps regularize circulation. Use 1 oz to 2 oz of plant per quart of water to prepare infusions.

Olive helps lower blood pressure and dilates peripheral arteries, especially in cases of hypertension related to atherosclerosis or anxiety. It is also a diuretic that has a beneficial effect on the kidneys. Use decoctions: Boil six or seven leaves in a cup of water for five minutes; drink three cups a day.

Nettle is a depurative that combats liver problems and hypertension. Boil 2 oz of leaves for two minutes, or 1 oz of roots for five minutes, in a quart of water; remove from heat and infuse for 10 minutes; drink three cups a day.

Apples help fight hypertension, especially when related to a liver or kidney lesion, accompanied by reduced urine flow. Rich in pectin, apples also help lower cholesterol levels. Because this fruit contains little sugar, it is ideal for diabetics. To prepare infusions, powder some dried peel (use organic apples that contain no pesticides) and add a tablespoon to a cup of boiling water; let stand for five minutes and drink a cup morning and night.

Buckwheat is a vasodilator that tones and strengthens blood vessels. Use 1 oz to 2 oz per quart of water to prepare infusions and drink three cups a day.

Linden is a hypotensor that helps lower blood pressure. It also has an antispasmodic and sedative effect that can help cure kidney and liver problems. Use 1 oz to 2 oz per quart of water to prepare infusions and drink three cups a day.

✐ High Cholesterol

Heart disease lesson number 1: Cholesterol is not the bad guy. That's right. In fact, it's perfectly normal to have a certain amount of cholesterol in your body. Your body needs cholesterol to function properly.

Problems arise, however, when you have too much of a certain kind of cholesterol (LDL, or *low density lipoproteins*) circulating in your system, resulting in accumulations of fatty deposits in arteries, which in turn cause various diseases like arteritis, atherosclerosis, diabetes, and high blood pressure, not to mention obesity.

Initial symptoms of a high cholesterol level include ringing in the ears, especially in the morning, spotted vision, feelings of heaviness, and a pins-and-needles sensation in the extremities. If you are experiencing these symptoms, you should consult a doctor.

Lifestyle

Move around as much as possible to promote better circulation and try to practice some breathing exercises every day. Research has also shown that there is a definite link between tension and cholesterol levels, which is why relaxation techniques and spending time in a calm, tranquil environment, removed from day-to-day worries, are helpful for people suffering from high cholesterol.

Also try to adhere to a regular schedule as much as possible, and cut down on cigarette smoking, which hardens arteries.

Nutrition

A hypotoxic diet is recommended for persons whose cholesterol level is slightly higher than normal. For those who have much too much cholesterol, a diet composed entirely of natural brown rice, white cheese, and salad can do wonders to regenerate blood vessels and reduce hypertension.

On the other hand, game meat, offal, blood pudding, brains, sweetbreads, meat from young animals, egg yolks, shellfish, sardines, anchovies, eels, beef fat, lard, butter, fresh cream, and fat cheese are all very rich in cholesterol.

The short version is: Try to avoid heavy meals containing a lot of animal fat, eggs, and dairy products. Eat more fish and less meat. Alcohol should be consumed in moderate amounts and certainly not with every meal. Liqueurs should be enjoyed only on special occasions.

Also reduce your intake of sugar, bread, pasta, and other starchy foods. Use non-hydrogenated sunflower seed, sesame seed or linseed oil for cooking and to season salads. Take wheat germ oil on a regular basis.

Plant Power

The natural world offers some excellent remedies for taming the cholesterol lion. Here are some of the most effective.

Artichokes are excellent for the liver, which is where cholesterol is produced in the body. Unfortunately, artichoke infusions (a pinch per cup of boiled water, three times a day, 15 minutes before meals) have a very bitter taste. You can buy the plant in tincture form in herbal and health food stores: 20 to 40 drops in a glass of water, three times a day, 15 minutes before meals. Or use the following preparation: 1 oz of artichoke leaves mixed with 2 oz of crushed dandelion roots and 1 oz of bittersweet flowers, boiled in a quart of water for 15 minutes; reheat a cup of the preparation every day, and use it to infuse 1 oz of hawthorn flowers and 1/2 oz of mistletoe leaves; take the remedy two days a week, sweetened with honey.

Birch is recommended for reducing high cholesterol levels. Pour a quart of boiling water over 2 oz of leaves and add a sprinkle of bicarbonate of soda when the temperature has dropped to about 100 degrees Fahrenheit; infuse for six hours, and drink four cups a day, between meals.

Rosemary is an excellent general stimulant, has a beneficial effect on the liver, and helps in the evacuation of bile. Soak two teaspoons of rosemary in a cup of water for two or three minutes, then bring to a boil for about 10 minutes. Drink two or three cups a day, before meals.

Speedwell soothes intestinal problems and alleviates stomach aches. In some cases it is also effective for reducing cholesterol levels. Add a teaspoon to a quart of boiling water and infuse for three minutes. Drink two cups a day.

❧ Hives

Hives are Mother Nature's way of telling you that you're allergic to something. Heed her warning, and avoid whatever you're allergic to. A second episode of hives can be dramatically worse than the first, and if they spread to the mouth and throat (a condition called Quincke's Edema), they can become life threatening.

The most common culprits for causing hives include shellfish, strawberries, pork, eggs, and cheese. If an outbreak of hives is accompanied by fever, which is usually not the case, consult a doctor.

Ideally you should identify the food, fiber, or other substance that seems to trigger attacks, and eliminate it, although doing so sometimes takes a lot of time and perseverance.

Liver problems, constipation, and even extremely cold or hot weather can also cause hives to appear on the skin.

General Care

Stay in bed during attacks and rub affected areas with lemon juice. Avoid using cosmetics (lipstick, blush, etc.), beauty creams, and nail polish. Also avoid aspirin, antibiotics, and quinine-based medications.

Nutrition

Drink only water for 24 hours. Then start taking some vegetable broth, and gradually wean yourself back onto solid food. Adopt a hypotoxic diet. You can also ingest some lime powder to alleviate symptoms. Foods to avoid include blue cheeses, foods rich in protein or nitrates, tomatoes, spices, wine, beer, and other alcoholic beverages.

Plant Power

For extreme cases of hives, see your doctor. But for mild, annoying cases, there are some effective home treatments, like the ones below, that you can use.

Burdock is often recommended for treating skin problems because of its diuretic and depurative effect. Crush some fresh leaves in a mortar and pestle, then soak them in pure olive oil for a day, in a sealed container; filter, press through a fine cloth, and apply locally to affected areas of skin. (Note that this remedy cannot be preserved for longer than a few days.)

Centaury is a depurative that combats attacks of hives related to liver problems or constipation. Infuse 1 oz of plant in a quart of water for 10 minutes; drink three cups a day for eight days.

Fumitory is a depurative that regulates liver functions. Use 1 oz per quart of water to prepare infusions (half the amount for children), and drink three or four cups a day for about a week.

Nettle is a diuretic and depurative that helps eliminate toxins. Boil 3 oz of leaves in a quart of water for 15 minutes; sip a teaspoon every hour.

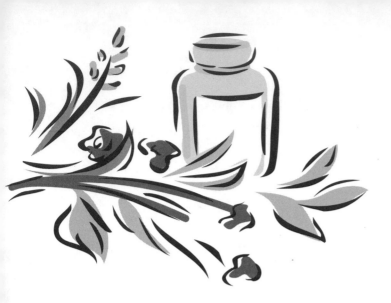

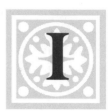

✐ Impetigo

Impetigo is a general term describing any of a number of skin diseases that shows up as an eruption of pustules. Most of these diseases are contagious and are caused by staphylococci bacteria. The initial infection, which occurs most often in children, is generally due to improper hygiene.

The symptoms are easy to spot. Pustules develop on the skin and eventually burst. Children scratch the crusts, causing open sores, which tend to fester in folds of the skin (under the armpits, behind the ears, on the neck, etc.).

General Care

Make sure children wash all parts of their body thoroughly. If lesions appear, cover affected areas with sterile compresses held in place with adhesive tape. This will prevent the infections from spreading.

To clean sores, use liquid soap or add a few drops of arnica tincture to some 45-proof alcohol. You can also disinfect lesions with mild peroxide to kill bacteria.

Nutrition

Drink 12 oz of fresh carrot juice (made from organic carrots if possible) every morning before breakfast, or towards the end of the afternoon. Cut down on fats, and have more fresh fruit, vegetables, fresh juices, etc. Meat should be boiled, grilled, or roasted.

Plant Power

Burdock is a depurative recommended for both internal and external use. To prepare decoctions, boil 2 oz in a quart of water for five minutes (for concentrated decoctions boil 7 oz in a quart of water for 10 minutes); filter and sweeten with a little honey. Use the ground roots or concentrated decoction for external treatments.

Birch is a diuretic that can be used internally or externally. For compresses add 2 oz of dried leaves to a quart of water and bring to a boil for three minutes. To prepare infusions, use 1 oz of leaves per quart of boiling water, and let stand for 10 minutes. In both cases add 1 gram of bicarbonate of soda when the temperature falls below 105 degrees Fahrenheit (in order to dissolve the plant's resin content).

Cabbage makes a very effective compress. Remove the large fibers, then flatten the leaves with a rolling pin and boil in milk for a few minutes. Or soak the leaves in lukewarm water for half a day. Apply directly to affected areas. You can do the same thing with carrots, although it's not so effective.

Walnut is a depurative and antibiotic. To prepare decoctions, add 1 oz of dried leaves to a quart of water and bring to a boil for five minutes, then remove from heat and let stand for 15 minutes; sweeten with honey and cool before drinking. Have three cups a day, between meals. Or you can sip a cup of the following herbal mixture in the morning before breakfast: 1 oz of dried walnut leaves, and 2/3 oz each of birch and sage leaves; infuse 1/3 oz in a cup of boiling water for 10 minutes.

Sage is an antiseptic fungicide (it destroys parasitic fungi) that accelerates healing of lesions and purifies the blood. Prepare infusions for internal use: 1 oz of sage per quart of boiling water; let stand for 10 minutes. For external use, prepare decoctions: Boil 3 oz of plant in a quart of water for 5 to 10 minutes.

Marigold is an anti-inflammatory and antiseptic that accelerates healing of lesions. Prepare decoctions for external use: Boil 1 oz of flowers in a quart of water for 10 minutes. You can also prepare your own marigold

THE FOODS OF LOVE

Certain foods, called aphrodisiacs, tend to stimulate sexual appetite. Some of the more common aphrodisiac foods include artichokes, onions, carrots, celery, lettuce, and oysters (because of their high zinc content). But don't expect to become sexually aroused after eating a couple of carrots! Adding more of these foods to your regular diet will have a subtle effect over an extended period of time.

A number of spices also enhance sexual desire, including coriander, cloves, and saffron. In fact, because odor is such an important part of sexuality, any spice or condiment that is pleasing to your sense of smell will have a positive effect on your sexual activity.

Finally, here are two of the world's most sensually stimulating teas to give your lovemaking a boost.

- **Aphrodisiac tea #1:** Mix the following ingredients: 1 oz of cow parsnip (or celery), 1 oz of savory, 1 oz of ginger, and a pinch of ginseng. Add two or three tablespoons of the mixture to a pint of water and simmer for 20 minutes. Drink three equal portions during the course of the day.
- **Aphrodisiac tea #2:** Combine 1 pinch of each of the following plants: grated nutmeg, sage, rosemary, oregano, chamomile, mint, juniper, and clove. Add the mixture to a quart of boiling water, let stand for 20 minutes, and drink a cup a day (the more you drink, the stronger the effect).

ointment to treat skin inflammation: Mix 2/3 oz of tincture with 1/4 cup of petroleum jelly (a ratio of one to nine) and apply to affected areas.

Impotence

Sexual impotence generally refers to the inability of a male either to become erect or to maintain an erection long enough to complete the act of sexual intercourse. If this happens more than 40 percent of the time, the impotence is considered chronic.

Factors like high cholesterol, low testosterone levels, obesity, diabetes, drug addiction, alcohol abuse, and certain conventional medications can all contribute to causing impotence.

Whatever the cause, it can become a frustrating and upsetting problem, both for the men who have it and for their sexual partners.

General Care

First consult with a urologist, and get a blood test. Three common caus-es of impotence (high cholesterol, diabetes, and low testosterone levels) can be diagnosed that way.

If you are obese and suffer from impotence, make an effort to lose weight. Tobacco and alcohol addiction also seem to have an adverse effect on sexual function.

If the problem is not physiological, it's emotional. Consult a qualified psychologist or sex therapist to help determine what the underlying mental problem might be (often a lack of self-esteem or confidence).

Lifestyle

Developing a sexual problem, like developing a disease, is a signal from the body, telling you that something is wrong. For example, you shouldn't be surprised to find yourself incapable of having sexual relations if you have been working much too hard, or spending night after night out on the town, drinking and eating to excess. In such cases all you have to do is give your body a chance to get back in sync with its natural cycle, and try not to abuse it in the future.

Because the human mind and body are interconnected in subtle ways, psychological factors like anxiety or stress can also result in sexual break-downs. The important thing is to listen to what your body is saying and take appropriate steps to eliminate any harmful habits you may have.

Plant Power

Cultures the world over have traditionally used herbs to improve sexual function. Combining the ones suggested below with lots of fresh air and moderate exercise may be just the thing you need to put the pizzazz back into your love life.

Cow parsnip has a tonic and stimulating effect on your entire organism, similar to that of ginseng, which is known to enhance sexual function. Use 1/2 oz of leaves per quart of boiling water to prepare your infusions. For extractions use 1/2 oz of roots and seeds per quart of water, and boil for 15 minutes.

Celery may have a rather bland taste and unexciting reputation, but it's known to have a positive effect on sexuality. To benefit fully from its aphrodisiac properties, drink fresh celery juice. This plant is especially beneficial for persons whose sexual function has been affected by disease, or who are recovering from a prolonged illness. Drink a teaspoon of freshly pressed juice an hour before meals. You can also mix celery juice with carrot and apple juice (use more carrot and apple than celery juice in your mix, because of celery's high sodium content).

Damiana has a pertinent scientific name: *Turnera aphrodisiaca*. The plant, which is native to Mexico and California, is reputed to be a powerful aphrodisiac and is particularly effective in cases where sexual problems are related to emotional or psychological disorders, mild depression, or extreme fatigue. To prepare infusions, use a pinch of dried leaves in one cup of boiling water and infuse for 15 minutes. You can also use a maceration: Soak 1/3 oz of leaves in a pint of water overnight. In both cases take one or two cups a day, and expect to wait about 10 days for results.

Ginger has a stimulating effect on the genital organs. Simply use it as a spice on a regular basis, either to cook with, or grated on salads, fruit, etc. Prepare infusions by pouring a cup of boiling water over half a teaspoon of powdered ginger mixed with a teaspoon of honey (you can add a little brandy if you like).

Ginseng is a well-known aphrodisiac. Use dried Korean ginseng root (Panax Ginseng) to prepare infusions: 1/2 oz per quart of boiling water; let stand for 10 minutes.

Savory is a tonic for both the mind and body. Use 2 oz per quart of boiling water to prepare your infusions, and drink a cup after meals.

❧ Infection

When laughter becomes infectious, we appreciate it. Anything else—bacteria, viruses, or fungi—is a problem.

So how do you know if you have an infection? In many cases, you'll develop a fever. If the infection is in the skin, you may have pustules or an area that's red and painful. The same is true of the throat. If you have a lung infection, you'll probably have a cough and possibly dark green or black mucous. In the urinary tract, you'll most likely feel a burning sensation. And in the digestive system, you may have heartburn, swelling, cramps, or nausea.

NATURE'S ANTISEPTICS

The antiseptic properties of plants have been known to people since pre-historic times and constitute one of the most important ways nature has benefited humankind. You can use these plants to fight infection, without any of the inconveniences of chemical antibiotics. Regular use of natural antibiotics is first and foremost a preventive measure, helping your organism become more resistant to disease.

- **Yarrow** is known to combat a number of types of infection. You can use it externally as a treatment for cuts and wounds (see page 87) or internally, as an infusion: Use 1/2 oz of plant per quart of boiling water, and let stand for 10 minutes.
- **Garlic** does a lot more than add flavor to foods—its antiseptic properties are, in fact, widely known. Garlic helps prevent infectious illnesses like the flu, diphtheria, infectious diarrhea, typhoid, bronchitis, emphysema, and tuberculosis. When added to your food, it disinfects your intestines without destroying your intestinal flora. Some experts suggest that eating garlic helps prevent stomach cancer. Make it a habit to add raw garlic to your salads, sauces, cooked vegetables, etc.
- **Elder** is a treatment of choice for persons suffering from respiratory infections. Prepare infusions with 1 oz of roots per quart of boiling water; let stand for 10 minutes and drink a cup before meals.
- **Sage** is primarily used as an external application. Prepare sage extractions by soaking 60 grams of leaves in a quart of water for 15 minutes; add some vinegar to obtain an antiseptic lotion.
- **Nasturtium** contains substances that make it a powerful antibiotic agent. There are various ways you can use this plant: added to salads, it helps strengthen your resistance to infectious disease; nasturtium juice (half a cup of fresh juice per day) can be used as both an internal and external disinfectant; taken in capsule form, nasturtium acts as an antibiotic that doesn't destroy your natural intestinal flora.

Plant Power

Nature has been kind in providing us with a whole arsenal of natural antibiotics. Here are some of the most useful.

Elecampane contains an antibacterial agent that is recommended for the treatment of respiratory infections. Prepare infusions using 1 oz of dried roots per quart of boiling water.

THE TROUBLE WITH ANTIBIOTICS

Although antibiotics can be extremely helpful in certain cases, they do present a number of disadvantages which you should be aware of.

First, there is the question of abuse. Antibiotics have become a kind of cure-all for minor ailments. But we're beginning to learn that too many antibiotics can actually be harmful to health and lead to problems like allergies, vertigo, deafness, and internal hemorrhaging.

Second, antibiotics destroy beneficial as well as harmful bacteria—notably your intestinal flora—making you more vulnerable to attack from harmful microbes like staphylococcus, streptococcus, and colon bacillus, not to mention yeast and fungus. So it's important to use antibiotics only when they are really needed. For most minor problems, plants offer a viable alternative.

To compensate for the loss of beneficial bacteria after using antibiotics, take brewer's yeast (available in liquid form, packaged in vials). Because brewer's yeast cells are not destroyed by antibiotic medications, they proliferate in your digestive tract and stop the spread of harmful microbes, which is a great help when you're recovering from an illness. Yogurt is also excellent for restoring intestinal flora and destroying harmful bacteria.

Lavender is a powerful antiseptic that is especially recommended for bronchial infections. To prepare decoctions, boil 1 oz in a quart of water for five minutes, then remove from heat and let stand for 10 minutes.

Papaya is an exotic fruit, available in some supermarkets, that contains an enzyme that combats external infections. Simply place a slice over the affected area to draw out pus.

Rose is recommended for sore throats, inflammation of the mouth or digestive system, runny noses, and bronchial infections. Its antiseptic properties help combat staphylococcus, colibacillus, proteus bacteria (found in the digestive and respiratory systems), and pyocyanic bacteria, which is responsible for infections in newborn infants or patients after certain surgical procedures. For sore throats, prepare concentrated infusions using 2 oz of petals per quart of water; drink two or three cups per day. To treat sores that are full of pus, use rose vinegar: Soak 3 oz of rose petals in white vinegar for 10 days in a glass container in direct sunlight or near some other heat source; apply directly to affected areas.

Thyme is an antiseptic balm that helps cure infections in the throat and breathing passages and minor infections of the intestinal and urinary tracts. It can also be used externally to treat infected cuts and burns. For digestive and respiratory infections, drink three cups of infusion per day, before meals: 1 oz of leaves and flowers per quart of water. You can also take 20 drops of essence of thyme per day, available in pharmacies and in herbal and health food stores. For throat infections: Add 2/3 oz of thyme to a quart of cold water; heat and boil for five minutes; filter, sweeten with a little honey, and use as a gargle.

∾ Insect Bites

Bees, wasps, hornets, and ants kill more people each year in the United States than either spiders or poisonous snakes. The reported number of fatalities is about 100 cases annually, but the actual number may be much higher.

FIRST AID FOR STINGS

If you notice swelling around the mouth or genitals, if hives begin to appear, if you have difficulty breathing or feel faint, call for emergency care immediately! But if the reaction is limited to local redness, pain, and swelling, you can treat the problem yourself.

If you're stung by a honey bee, you'll have to remove the stinger from your skin. Other types of bees and wasps don't leave their stingers behind. The venom sac attached to the stinger can take up to three minutes to empty, so getting it out quickly reduces pain. *Don't use your fingers!* You may end up squeezing the remaining venom from the sack. Instead, use the edge of a credit card to scrape it out.

If you have no other remedies available, you can apply a temporary lotion composed of a mixture of salted water and vinegar or of water and baking soda.

Leek, marigold, or parsley can be used as a first-aid treatment. Chew the plant until it turns to pulp in your mouth, then apply directly to the bite. Leek leaves can also be crushed between your fingers to extract the sap, which you then apply to the bite.

Rubbing the bite with a slice of onion will help alleviate pain.

Most people will respond to the sting of an insect with a little redness, pain, and swelling around the wound. But 1 in 100 of us will have a much more violent reaction, called anaphylactic shock, which causes more general swelling, especially in the throat, where breathing can become blocked.

If after a sting you become lightheaded or nauseated or if you break out in hives, have difficult breathing or swallowing, or notice your voice getting hoarse, you need to get emergency medical treatment as soon as possible.

Death among allergic people has been known to occur within five minutes of a sting, so time is of the essence.

Lifestyle

Some of these simple precautions can help you avoid getting stung in the first place.

Use covers. Make sure to cover any food or trash you bring outside, so that bees won't be attracted to it.

Stay alert. Keep an eye peeled for bee or wasp nests when you're out of doors. Remember, they can be anywhere from the eaves of a house to a hole in the ground.

Wear shoes. When you're walking in grass, weeds, or among flowers, bees can be hard to see. You don't want to step on one accidentally. You might even want to clear your lawn of dandelions and clover, which attract honey bees.

Don't swat. If a bee lands on you, don't slap it against your body. First, it might sting you before it dies. More important, its crushed body will give off a pheromone (chemical scent) that signals other bees or wasps to swarm and attack. Shoo the bee away with one sweep of your hand and walk calmly to a sheltered place.

Plant Power

If you have a simple, local reaction to an insect sting or bite, there are some excellent plant remedies to stop pain and help healing.

Blackcurrant can be applied directly to a bite to alleviate pain and soothe inflammation. Rub leaves together to extract the sap and apply to the bite.

Lavender is an antiseptic that promotes healing. For insect bites, rub leaves together to extract the sap and apply directly to the bite. Or apply a decoction: 1 oz per quart of boiling water. Lavender oil is another alternative (this has to be prepared in advance). Soak 3 oz of lavender, 2 oz of St. John's wort flower tops, and 1 oz of chamomile in half a quart of 90-proof alcohol for 15 days; filter, add 1/3 oz of camphor and a third of a quart of water; shake well before applying.

Plantain soothes pain caused by insect bites: Simply rub fresh leaves over the affected area.

Savory helps calm irritation caused by insect bites. Crush some fresh plant and apply as a poultice to the affected area.

Sage helps alleviate insect bite pain: Use crushed leaves as a poultice.

⇒ Insomnia

Rip Van Winkle slept for 20 years. Ever wonder what made him so tired? It wasn't a sleeping pill, that's for sure. It's common knowledge that sleeping pills provide only temporary relief for insomnia, inducing an unnatural sleep that interrupts the regular dream cycle. They can actually do more harm than good over the long run—they contain toxins that can damage the kidneys and liver and have an adverse affect on your state of mind.

Lifestyle

If you want to sleep at night, get up and move during the day. A sedentary lifestyle deprives the body of opportunities to expend energy through movement. In other words, it leaves you with your motor still revving at the end of the day. Fatigue generated by some simple form of physical activity can often solve the problem of insomnia quickly, safely, and effectively.

Ideal Sleeping Conditions

Your bedroom should be well ventilated, especially if you sleep with another person. Temperature should be kept at about 60 degrees Fahrenheit. Avoid potentially stimulating discussions or intense intellectual activity just before going to bed.

Some people are very sensitive to sound. If you have a problem falling asleep because of ambient noise, try using car plugs (available in pharmacies). The only downside is that you might become addicted to them and not be able to sleep without them.

SEDATIVE PLANTS

These plants have a calming effect on the nervous system. One of the great advantages of plants, as opposed to synthetic medications, is that while they are highly effective, they are far less toxic. Choose the plant remedy that suits your needs best from the following list:

- **Hawthorn** is helpful for treating nervous disorders like insomnia, irritability, palpitations, and so on. Drink two or three cups of hawthorn infusion for a period of 10 days every month. To prepare infusions, use 1/2 oz of flowers per quart of boiling water.
- **Horehound** (also known as black hemp nettle) is an antispasmodic that helps alleviate all types of nerve-related problems (palpitations, anxiety, hot flashes, agitated sleep). Take three or four teaspoons of hawthorn tincture per day. Preparation: Soak one heaping cup of the plant in two cups of eau-de-vie or brandy for 15 days; filter and store in an airtight container.
- **Common chamomile,** also called Rumanian chamomile, is an antispasmodic that calms frayed nerves and helps alleviate pain. Drink two or three cups of chamomile infusion per day. Use 1 oz of leaves per quart of water.
- **Marshmallow** is an emollient (i.e., it has a soothing, softening effect on surface tissues). Drink three cups of infusion per day. Preparation: 1 oz of leaves and flowers per quart of water. For external applications (as compresses), prepare an extraction: 1 oz per quart of water.
- **Hops** have a calming effect on the nervous system and can be used as a tranquilizer or sleeping potion. Drink two cups of infusion per day, between meals. Preparation: 1/2 oz of cones per quart of water.
- **Valerian** can be used to calm the nervous system and promote sleep. Don't drink more than one or two cups of infusion per day (if you take more, the plant's effects will be reversed and you will become more nervous instead of calm) and only for a short period of time (about a week). Prepare extractions using 1 oz to 2 oz of dried roots per quart of water. Add hops, passion flower, or linden to improve the slightly unpleasant taste.

Nutrition

Avoid copious meals shortly before bedtime, as a full stomach can prevent you from sleeping. You should obviously also avoid stimulants like coffee or tea in the evening. Drink some kind of sedative infusion instead. Or else try a bowl of yogurt sweetened with honey. If you wake up in the middle of the night, try eating just a teaspoon of honey.

Food combinations are also important: Meat, egg, or cheese dishes (containing a lot of nitrates) or concentrated vegetable dishes like soup or steamed vegetables (which contain a lot of minerals) can cause insomnia. Lettuce, on the other hand, is an excellent sedative.

Plant Power

The plants listed below are mild sedatives that are not likely to become addictive.

Sweet woodruff fortifies and calms the nervous system and helps fight the blues when used for an extended period of time. It works for both children and adults. Prepare infusions using 1 oz to 2 oz per quart of water, and drink three or four cups a day.

Hawthorn has a sedative and antispasmodic effect on the cardiovascular system. It also helps alleviate nervousness, anxiety, and nocturnal fears in children. Boil 1/3 oz of crushed plant in a quart of water for three minutes, then remove from heat and let stand for 10 minutes.

Black hemp nettle (also called black horehound) is recommended for persons who are anxious or stressed. It also alleviates anxiety and palpitations. Use 1 oz to 2 oz per quart of water to prepare infusions, and drink two cups during the course of the day, and one before going to bed. Because of the bitter taste, some people prefer taking this plant in tincture form: Soak one part plant in two parts eau-de-vie or brandy for 15 days. When it's ready, take two or three teaspoons during the course of the day.

Chamomile promotes sleep, facilitates digestion, and regulates menstrual flow. Prepare infusions using 1 oz per quart of water and drink a cup a half hour before or after meals. You can also try the following mixture: 2 oz of ladies mantle, 1 oz of hawthorn, and 1 oz of chamomile flowers.

Hops have a mild tranquilizing effect that calms the nervous system and promotes sleep. Prepare infusions using 1/2 oz to 1 oz of cones per quart of boiling water; let stand for 10 minutes, and sweeten with a little honey.

Lotus should be used with care because of its cyanhydric acid content. The plant has a sedative, mildly narcotic effect and is recommended for cases of insomnia linked to anxiety. Anxious persons will actually find the plant slightly euphoric and enjoy a calm, regenerating sleep, allowing them to awaken feeling refreshed instead of tired. Prepare infusions using 2 oz to 3 oz of the whole plant (the flowers contain more cyanhydric acid than other parts) per quart of water; let stand for 10 minutes. Drink a cup around 10 in the morning, and another before going to bed, for a maximum of 10 consecutive days, then stop for at least 10 days.

Lemon balm is a sedative, antispasmodic, and stimulant. It has a beneficial effect on people who are nervous, irritable, over-excited, or depressed and acts as a natural tranquilizer or tonic, depending on the case. Prepare infusions using 2/3 oz of flower tops per quart of water and drink three or four cups a day.

Orange has a calming, sedative effect on the nervous system. It also helps alleviate headaches and stomach aches. Use 1/2 oz of leaves or flowers per quart of water to prepare infusions.

Passion flower calms the nervous system and helps alleviate anxiety and stress related to work, both of which can cause insomnia. Drink a couple of cups of infusion to enjoy normal, regenerating sleep.

Linden relaxes the mind and body and helps alleviate mental agitation that can disturb sleep. Use it in conjunction with hawthorn or passion flower, in infusion form.

Valerian alleviates various types of nerve-related problems, including insomnia. It helps dispel fears, obsessions, phobias, etc. Drink two cups of maceration per day. To prepare a maceration, soak 1/3 oz of fresh valerian in some water overnight; sweeten with honey, and mix with a verbena, orange, or mint infusion. You can also take 10 to 20 drops of tincture, mixed with another herbal infusion (hawthorn, verbena, orange, or mint). To prepare the tincture, soak 7 oz of fresh chopped roots in a quart of eau-de-vie or brandy for 15 days.

❧ Intestinal Parasites

The very thought of parasites can make us shudder, but the fact is, kids get them all the time in the form of small round worms that establish themselves in the small intestine, caecum (a part of the large intestine), and the appendix. That's right; we're talking about pinworms.

These parasites cause intense anal itching, which children find particularly unpleasant. Unable to prevent themselves from scratching, they soon spread the infestation to other parts of the body.

There are, of course, other kinds of intestinal parasites, and all need to be looked after. Symptoms may include disturbed sleep, facial pallor, digestive problems, acute appendicitis (if the parasites penetrate the appendix), nightmares, nocturnal grinding of teeth, nervousness, irritability, melancholy, difficulty urinating, and even vision problems.

TOP FIVE WAYS TO PREVENT INTESTINAL PARASITES

- Avoid eating raw meat (steak tartar) or fish unless you are absolutely sure the product has been tested and approved.
- Cook pork meat for at least half an hour.
- Wash fruit and vegetables that have been grown with chemical fertilizers very carefully.
- Use lots of chives, garlic, and wild garlic when you cook.
- Keep your pets from licking you. Household pets can spread parasites. Although pet lovers may not like to hear this, being licked by a dog or cat is sometimes the cause of parasitic (tenia) infestation.

Nutrition

The food you eat can be a source of contamination, which is why you should be very careful about the kinds of foods you buy and cook.

Eating raw carrots before breakfast and a quarter of an hour before your midday and evening meals, as well as ingesting lots of garlic, pineapple or raw cabbage, will help prevent or eliminate intestinal parasites.

General Care

Before undergoing conventional treatments, try the medicinal plant remedies below, especially with children, who are less able to tolerate toxic medications.

During treatment, rigorous hygiene is essential, especially for children who tend to scratch their anus and then put their fingers in their mouth, causing repeated infestations. Make sure both the bedroom and bedclothes of the infected individual are as clean as possible, and cut the nails of children very short so that eggs won't lodge under them.

Garlic kills some intestinal worms (and increases sperm count in males!) according to the Talmud. Boil one or two cloves in 7 oz of milk and drink a couple of cups a day.

Gentian is a depurative that stimulates bile secretions and helps combat parasites.

German chamomile can be used as a general remedy for all types of parasites. Prepare infusions using 1 pinch per quart of boiling water.

Onions help kill parasites, notably a type called *ascaris*. You can simply eat them or, for one week of the month, drink a glass a day of this onion-alcohol brew: Soak some raw finely chopped onion in an equal weight of alcohol for 10 days; add two teaspoons to half a glass of sweetened water.

Pumpkin helps eliminate tapeworm and several roundworms, like *oxyuris*, that affect children. To combat oxyuris, adults should ingest 20 to 30 pumpkin seeds (children should eat between 10 and 15 seeds). Remove seeds from their shell without removing the greenish membrane covering the seed itself. Chew the seeds well, and take a teaspoon of castor oil an hour later. To treat tapeworm, be very careful about your diet, and ingest 80 to 100 pumpkin seeds per day, four times a day, making sure to chew them well. Once again, take a teaspoon of castor oil an hour after eating the seeds. If your initial attempt to get rid of the parasites does not work, try it again, because there is no danger of harmful side effects.

Thyme is safe for children. Use infusions (1 oz per quart of water) or essence of thyme: three to five drops on a cube of sugar, twice a day.

Wild thyme kills parasites. Use 2/3 oz per quart of water to prepare infusions and drink three or four cups a day.

Valerian combats parasites, soothes convulsions in children, and promotes sleep. Soak 1/3 oz of fresh valerian root in some water overnight; sweeten with honey and mix with a verbena, orange, or mint infusion; drink two cups per day. You can also take 10 to 20 drops of valerian tincture at night before going to bed, mixed with another herbal infusion (hawthorn, verbena, orange, or mint): Soak 7 oz of fresh, chopped roots in a quart of eau-de-vie or brandy for 15 days. Note that it is important to respect the recommended doses, as this plant can have an adverse effect if abused.

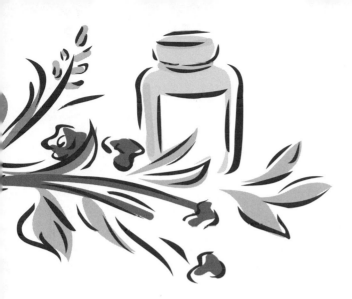

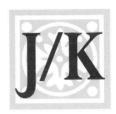

🌿 Kidney Problems

The two most common ailments you're likely to encounter where the kidneys are concerned are inflammation (nephritis) and stones.

Nephritis is usually caused by an infection of some kind. In some cases the problem arises after a bout of angina, sinusitis, or scarlet fever caused by streptococcus bacteria. Symptoms include high fever, dark-colored urine (because of its high albumin content), and difficulty urinating. Medical treatment is essential.

The formation of kidney stones has a lot to do with dietary habits. Drinking too much tea, eating too much meat or cheese, not drinking enough water, or even a vegetarian diet containing excessive amounts of green vegetables can all result in the formation of a stone. Attacks occur while the stone passes from the kidney into the urethra. Symptoms include difficulty urinating, bloody urine, and severe pain in the kidneys and/or bladder.

Plant Power

Many of the plant remedies recommended for gallstones will also work for kidney stones. Here are a few more that will help you through the rough spots, as well as some that are good for nephritis.

MY DOCTOR SAYS I HAVE ALBUMINARIA. WHAT IS IT?

This disorder, characterized by an inflammation of the kidneys, is caused by an excess of a blood protein called albumin. It's often associated with nephritis and can be either acute or chronic (chronic cases are more diffi-cult to diagnose). Symptoms of acute albuminuria include shivering, fever, severe headaches, and vomiting. Urination becomes difficult and infrequent, and the urine is usually very dark. Eyelids, ankles, legs, and other bodily tis-sues become swollen, and pressing the swelling with a finger leaves a pit.

In cases of chronic albuminaria, you tend to urinate often. Other symp-toms include headaches, generalized pain, muscular cramps, dizziness, and ringing in the ears, all caused by a compound called urea accumulating in the kidneys, preventing them from filtering the blood as they normally do.

Persons suffering from acute albuminaria should suspend their normal activities and remain in bed. Intestines should be flushed (using an enema), and the kidneys wrapped in flannel and kept warm. Diet should be restrict-ed to water sweetened with lactose (2 oz of lactose per quart of water, taken in small quantities throughout the day).

For cases of chronic albuminaria, get a lot of sleep, keep your kidneys warm by wrapping some flannel around your waist, avoid cold and extreme temperature changes, and don't overdo things as far as physical or intellec-tual effort is concerned.

Only a specialist can diagnose whether the problem is acute or chronic, and recommend an appropriate treatment (dialysis, or even a kidney trans-plant in very serious cases).

Borage is recommended for cases of acute nephritis accompanied by edema. Its soothing, diuretic effect stimulates kidney activity. Use 1 oz of flowers per quart of water to prepare infusions and drink three or four cups a day.

Horsetail is a powerful diuretic that helps combat kidney disorders, including nephritis. Boil 2 oz of dried plant in a quart of water for half an hour, and drink three or four cups a day.

Elder is a depurative, diuretic, and laxative recommended for cases of nephritis accompanied by edema. Use decoctions: Boil 2 oz of elder in a quart of water until half the water has evaporated. Drink small amounts throughout the course of the day.

Broom heather acts as an antiseptic and diuretic on the urinary tract and is one of the ingredients of a herbal remedy for kidney stones: 1 oz of broom heather, 1 oz of couchgrass, 2 oz of pellitory-of-the-wall, and 1 oz of horsetail; infuse 1/3 oz of the mixture in a quart of boiled water for half an hour and drink four or five cups a day.

Cherry is a diuretic: Soak 7 oz of cherry stems in a quart of water for 12 hours, then bring to a boil for 10 minutes; drink half a quart per day. To add taste, you can pour the boiling infusion over some dried cherries.

Fennel is a diuretic that facilitates digestion and helps prevent the formation of kidney stones. Boil a handful of wattle (the feathery part of the peel) in a quart of water for a minute or two, then add two teaspoons of fennel seeds.

Juniper has long been used as a diuretic to help treat kidney stones and bladder inflammation. It also has an antiseptic effect. Do not, however, use juniper as a cure for an extended period of time, as the plant will eventually irritate the stomach. Use 1 oz per quart of water to prepare infusions.

Pellitory has a diuretic, soothing effect, and can be used both internally and externally. Prepare infusions with 1 oz of fresh plant per quart of water, and drink two or three cups a day between meals. You can also extract the juice and take three to five teaspoons a day. For compresses, prepare a concentrated infusion: 2 oz of fresh plant per quart of water; soak some strips of cotton in the infusion and apply to the kidney region; hold in place (for half an hour) with a flannel bandage.

Parsley is a diuretic and tonic recommended for the treatment of urinary and kidney problems. Drink a tablespoon of juice in the morning before breakfast or a cup of infusion before meals. Use an extractor to obtain your juice, or grind some fresh parsley in a mortar and pestle, add a little water, and squeeze through a fine cloth. To prepare infusions, use a handful of fresh plant per quart of water.

Horsetail is a diuretic that helps eliminate kidney stones. It also helps re-mineralize the body. Add 1 1/2 to 2 oz of horsetail to a quart of cold water, boil for 30 minutes, then remove from heat and let stand for 10 minutes. Drink a cup in the morning and another in the early afternoon.

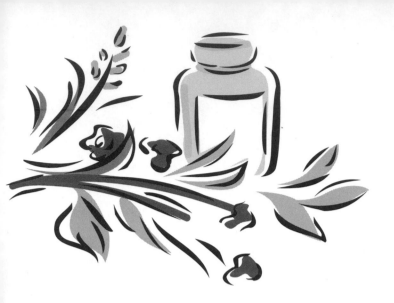

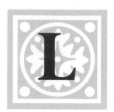

🍃 Laryngitis

It's the nightmare of every opera diva: She opens her mouth and nothing comes out but a breathy squeak. Better she should pass out in the middle of a performance!

It can happen to anyone. All it takes is a little inflammation of the larynx (the voice box in your throat) to cause partial or total extinction of the voice.

Acute laryngitis sometimes comes with fever, dry coughing, itching in the throat, and lots of mucus. It usually occurs after catching a cold.

Chronic laryngitis, on the other hand, does not cause fever or coughing, so if your voice remains hoarse for longer than two weeks, consult a doctor.

General Care

In acute cases it's best not to use your voice until the inflammation is gone. Don't smoke, and avoid hot damp rooms. Inhalations of eucalyptus, mint, etc. are effective.

For severe cases, especially those affecting children, wrap the neck in hot compresses, keep the child warm, and make sure that breathing passages are free of obstruction.

Plant Power

With the right plant remedy, you can speed up the return of your voice to its natural, full tone. Try these.

Hedge mustard acts as an antispasmodic on breathing passages and can help restore a voice that has been silenced by laryngitis. Infuse 2⁄3 oz of dried plant in a quart of boiling water for 20 minutes and drink three or four cups a day. This plant is

> ## HEDGE MUSTARD SYRUP
>
> **N**ot all remedies have to be bitter. Here's a recipe for a sweet syrup using hedge mustard: Boil 1 oz of hedge mustard in a quart of water until one third of the water has evaporated; add 1⁄3 oz of licorice and heat in a double boiler until it dissolves; filter and add 6 oz to 7 oz of honey; place in a heat-proof container and heat until the liquid turns to syrup.

also recommended for persons whose professions tend to strain their voice (actors, singers, public speakers, etc.). Drink three cups a day (one just before performance time).

Malva is an emollient (it relaxes tissues) that helps soothe inflammation of the larynx and relieves the dryness in the throat that often accompanies the condition. Boil 2⁄3 oz of flowers in a quart of water for five minutes; drink three or four cups a day or use as a gargle. To prepare compresses, use the same herbal decoction, reheated in a little water, and mix in some barley flour; spread the paste on some cotton or linen while still hot and wrap the throat; leave the compress in place overnight if possible.

Bitter milkwort helps soothe irritated throats. To prepare decoctions, boil 6 oz of roots in a quart of water for 10 minutes.

Liver Problems

A healthy liver is indispensable for the proper functioning of your body. The liver purifies the blood, retaining certain nutrients, eliminating waste and toxins, and replenishing the blood with substances needed for metabolism. It also controls the assimilation of lipids and the storage of important nutrients such as glycogen (glucose), vitamins, and minerals.

There are many types of liver disorders, giving rise to diseases like hepatitis and cirrhosis. A liver malfunction can also cause symptoms in other

WHEN THE LIVER CRIES OUT FOR HELP

It may be easier than you think to trace an ailment to the liver. Here's what to look for:

- Your liver (situated on the right side of your abdomen) is swollen and sensitive to the touch.
- You feel an aching pain in your abdomen, and your skin is yellowish (characteristic symptoms of jaundice).
- Veins in the skin covering your abdomen are dilated.
- You suffer from lack of appetite, nausea, and vomiting.
- The whites of your eyes are yellowish, you feel very tired between meals, experience sensations of dizziness or itching, or develop hives.
- You are always thirsty, and you find fried or greasy foods, sweets, or oranges repulsive.

organs, including chronic constipation, difficult digestion, various skin problems (eczema, hives), headaches, migraines, and chronic fatigue.

The liver also acts as a link between your psychological state and your physical health. In other words, it is the liver's affect on metabolism that translates negative emotions into physical health problems.

Nutrition

We cannot overemphasize the importance of nutrition for preventing and curing liver problems. Our physical constitution is, to a large extent, inherited. But the degree of strain we place on our digestive system over the course of our lives is a matter of choice.

Next to consuming too much alcohol, perhaps the worst thing you can do for your liver is eat fatty foods. Even if you have a mild liver problem, you should reduce your fat intake as much as possible. Here are some ways to do that.

Get rid of the grease. Avoid greasy, fried, and dairy foods, especially meat, butter, and fatty cheeses.

Cook meat the no-fat way. Meat should be grilled, roasted, or steamed. Opt for lean fish instead of meat whenever possible.

Eat light and right. Make these foods staples of your diet: dried fruit (prunes, raisins, figs, etc.), green vegetables like spinach and watercress (cooked if possible), potatoes, carrots, sauerkraut, artichokes, celery, salads containing bitter plants like endive or dandelion, rice, whole grain bread, dried vegetables and bean yogurt, uncooked sunflower or sesame seed oil, brewer's yeast, and sesame seed in all its forms.

Plant Power

Medicinal plants are a great way to treat liver problems. Nevertheless, it is important to consult a physician and obtain a professional diagnosis if you suspect your liver is giving you trouble.

Agrimony is a diuretic recommended for the extended treatment of chronic liver problems and jaundice. The plant also tones the digestive tract and helps cure various kidney disorders, including kidney stones. Prepare infusions using 2 oz to 3 oz of whole plant per quart of water and drink a few cups a day. Agrimony can also be combined with bedstraw and sweet woodruff (3 oz each); drink a cup in the morning before breakfast and two more during the course of the day, taking small sips.

Artichoke is excellent for regenerating the liver and regulating liver functions. The plant is often recommended for treating liver and gallbladder problems. Because artichoke decoctions are very bitter, it might be best to buy the extract or tincture, available in health food stores and pharmacies. Take 0.6 grams of extract (which is very active) per day, or 20 to 30 drops of tincture three times a day, about a quarter of an hour before meals.

LIVER ATTACKS

Characterized by severe pain on the right side of the stomach, these episodes are caused by spasms of the bile ducts, sometimes due to the presence of a gallstone.

Liver attacks accompanied by vomiting of bile are usually caused by appendicitis or a food or medication that the body cannot tolerate.

Attacks can also be psychosomatic, brought on by strong emotions. Sufferers generally seek darkness and feel nauseated, although no vomiting occurs.

If you—or someone close to you— suffer from any of the above symptoms, be sure to consult a qualified medical practitioner for an accurate diagnosis.

In the meantime, it's best not to eat anything for 24 hours. Drink water, mixed with a little milk curd or yogurt. The following day start drinking vegetable broth and/or fruit juice to rebuild strength.

Elecampine is a cholagogic plant (stimulates bile secretions) that strengthens sluggish intestines. It is recommended for the treatment of dry, seborrheic dermatitis or eczema related to a liver problem. Use 1 oz of roots per quart of water to prepare infusions and drink a cup before meals.

Boldo is a tonic that facilitates digestion and stimulates bile secretions. Use it with care, because it is mildly toxic. To prepare infusions, add 10 grams of leaves to a quart of boiled water along with a little mint to increase its effectiveness.

Celandine is beneficial for both the liver and gallbladder, and increases bile secretions. The plant is recommended for the treatment of cholecystitis, chronic jaundice, gallstones, chronic hepatitis, and cirrhosis. To prepare infusions, use 1/2 oz to 1 oz of dried leaves per quart of boiling water; remove from heat and let stand for ten minutes; drink one cup along with each meal of the day. To benefit from the plant's depurative effect, also helpful for curing liver disorders, take a teaspoon of fresh juice in the morning before breakfast.

Chicory purifies the blood, and acts as a cholagogic (stimulates bile secretions), a diuretic, and a mild laxative. It is recommended for the treatment of liver insufficiency, gallstones, jaundice, gallbladder engorgement, and liver and spleen congestion. Add chicory to your salads or prepare infusions using 2 oz of roots per quart of water. For maximum effectiveness, combine chicory with artichoke.

Couchgrass (also called doggrass) helps stimulate kidney functions and eliminate kidney stones. It is also recommended for cases of jaundice, liver and spleen congestion, gallstones, and liver insufficiency. Soak 1 oz of roots in a quart of water for a few hours and drink two or three cups a day.

Common broom is a diuretic that purifies the blood. It's good for the treatment of certain liver and gallbladder disorders, notably chronic hepatitis. Boil 1 oz to 2 oz of stems in a quart of water for 5 to 10 minutes, then remove from heat and let stand for 15 minutes. Drink five to six cups a day.

Gentian helps drain the liver and gallbladder and is recommended for liver disorders accompanied by digestive problems. Boil 1/2 oz to 2/3 oz of roots in a quart of water for 10 minutes, and drink a cup before meals.

Note: Do not use gentian every day, because it can cause headaches or nausea when ingested for extended periods of time.

Dandelion is a tonic and diuretic that helps clean out your organism. It's an excellent remedy for liver congestion and gallbladder problems. It increases bile secretions and is also recommended for cases of liver insufficiency, jaundice, and painful liver attacks. Use young leaves and stems in salads (in season) or drink four to six cups of dandelion infusion a day: Boil 2 oz in a quart of water for five minutes and sweeten with a little honey.

Black radish is recommended for persons suffering from cholecystitis and other liver disorders. It increases bile production, improves bladder functions, and cures gallstones. You can take a small amount of radish extract diluted in a little water in the morning before breakfast or eat some grated radish at the start of your meals. Fresh radish juice is best mixed with fresh carrot juice to prevent intestinal irritation.

Rosemary is a general tonic and stimulant and is recommended for cases of hepatitis, jaundice, liver congestion, and gallbladder inflammation. It also has a sedative effect and a very pleasant taste. Use 1 1/2 oz of dried leaves per quart of boiling water to prepare infusions; let stand for 15 minutes and drink four or five cups a day.

Sage has a beneficial effect on tired livers, acting as a tonic and stimulant. Use 2/3 oz per quart of boiling water to prepare infusions. Drink a cup after meals and one before going to bed.

Marigold is a depurative and is recommended for the treatment of infectious jaundice. Prepare decoctions using 2 oz per quart of water.

❧ Low Blood Pressure

Having low blood pressure (hypotension) is not necessarily a bad thing. It becomes a problem only when it's accompanied by chronic fatigue, dizziness, fainting (especially when you sit or stand abruptly), chronically cold extremities, or ringing in the ears.

Causes of the condition vary but can include physical injury, significant blood loss, or severe dehydration. Some medications (antidepressants or diuretics, for example) can also cause low blood pressure.

NATURE'S LITTLE PICK-ME-UP

Maybe it's why bees never get tired: Pollen, which is not a plant but a natural product derived from plants, can help alleviate fatigue due to low blood pressure. Take a teaspoon every morning along with your breakfast. Combined with marine algae, pollen also makes an excellent remedy for male impotence, which is often a side effect of low blood pressure.

Plant Power

When it comes to regulating blood pressure, plants pack plenty of power. Try some of the ones listed below to bring you up to speed.

Hawthorn is a natural fortifier that has a regulating and tonic effect on the heart. Its tranquilizing, antispasmodic properties produce no harmful side effects. Hawthorn lowers blood pressure, especially in cases of neuroarthritic hypertension, but it's also useful in treating hypotension (low blood pressure) and atherosclerosis. *Note, however, that this plant should not be used for an extended period of time, because it can inhibit normal heart and liver functions. To avoid these effects, all you have to do is stop taking the plant for a few days, say one week out of every month.* Boil 2 oz of flowers and berries in a quart of water for three minutes; drink three cups a day, three weeks per month.

Shepherd's purse regulates blood circulation and menstrual flow in women. To prepare infusions use 1 oz to 2 oz of dried plant per quart of boiling water and let stand for 10 minutes. Drink two cups per day until circulation returns to normal.

Milk thistle is a tonic that is effective for treating states of general fatigue or physical or mental exhaustion due to overwork or stress. It also has a tonic and regulating effect on the circulation and nervous systems. It is especially recommended for cases of hypotension accompanied by excessive perspiration and dizziness when switching abruptly from a seated to a standing position. Boil 3 oz of seeds in a quart of water for 15 minutes, then infuse for 10 minutes; drink three cups a day, before meals.

Sage is a fortifier and stimulant that is recommended for cases of low blood pressure, chronic fatigue, and nervous problems, or during periods of convalescence. Drink two or three cups of infusion per day.

✒ Lung Inflammation

Many seniors—even those who don't smoke—suffer from fits of coughing, especially in the early morning, accompanied by expectoration of white mucus. Medicinal plants can be very effective for treating this disorder.

Plant Power

Ground ivy makes an effective treatment for inflamed lungs. Prepare infusions using 1 oz per quart of boiling water and drink three or four cups a day.

Plantain helps alleviate coughing and soothes irritated breathing passages. Use the plant to prepare decoctions: Boil 1 oz to 2 oz of plantain in a quart of water for 10 minutes.

Milkwort reduces mucus secretions, stimulates digestion, and acts as a general tonic. To prepare decoctions, boil 5 oz of the plant in a quart of water for 10 minutes; sweeten with honey, and drink four cups a day between meals.

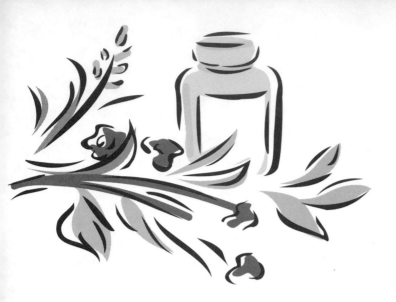

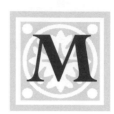

❧ Measles

First there are fever, tearing eyes and runny nose, sensitivity to light, and coughing. Then white spots appear inside the mouth; fever intensifies; and the neck, chest, stomach, and legs erupt with red spots. At this point, body temperature may rise to 103 degrees Fahrenheit. It's one of the great childhood scourges. It's the measles.

It may be tempting to ignore this disease, assuming it's just one of those things that all kids go through, but that would be a mistake. Measles can cause a number of complications, some of which are serious, including otitis, pharyngitis, and bronchial pneumonia.

Plant Power

If body temperature stays at 103 degrees for more than a day, contact your doctor. Plants are useful as complements to conventional medical or homeopathic treatments. They are especially effective for eliminating toxins and combating infection.

Garlic is an excellent remedy for contagious diseases, acting as a powerful antiseptic. Boil two or three large cloves of garlic in a glass of water or milk; drink one or two glasses a day. You can also prepare garlic syrup: Boil 2 oz of crushed garlic in a glass of water; filter and add 2 oz of honey; take two or three tablespoons a day. Another preparation consists of extracting

GERMAN MEASLES

Despite its reputation as a childhood disease, German measles (or rubella), which is spread by a virus, also affects women between the ages of 15 and 35. Eruptions mainly appear in folds of skin around joints—ankles, knees, wrists, and hands. These eruptions resemble those caused by measles and scarlet fever, but they disappear more rapidly. Once a person has contracted the disease, he or she is immune to further attacks for a long period of time.

If a woman contracts German measles during the second or third month of pregnancy, emergency medical treatment is an absolute must, because the disease can cause fetal malformations and other major problems. To prevent this, an immunizing vaccination is available, generally administered to girls before reaching school age. If you are pregnant and suspect you have rubella, see a doctor immediately for a precise diagnosis.

Although German measles eruptions usually disappear after three days, infected persons should be quarantined for a week to avoid the risk of contaminating others. Note that nasal secretions are the agent through which the disease is usually transmitted.

Although rubella and measles may look similar, they're caused by different viruses. To distinguish between the two, look for the following symptoms:

- An absence of fever when eruptions appear indicates that the problem is German measles.
- German measles is accompanied by inflammation behind the ears, on the neck, in the armpits, and around the groin.
- German measles doesn't cause white spots in the mouth, although the membranes on the inside of the cheeks are red.

the juice from a half pound of garlic and mixing it with an equal amount of 40-proof alcohol; take two or three teaspoons a day, 10 days out of every month, to avoid contracting an infectious disease.

Borage is recommended for cases of measles, scarlet fever, and chicken pox. The plant reduces fever, alleviates coughing, and stimulates elimination of toxins because of its diuretic effect. Use 1 oz to 2 oz of flowers per quart of boiled water to prepare infusions and take four cups a day.

Horehound stimulates expectoration, soothes coughing, and fights a large variety of infectious diseases. Use 1 oz of plant per quart of water to prepare infusions and drink three or four cups a day.

Onion is a diuretic, antiseptic, and antibiotic that also alleviates persistent coughing. Put 10 oz of raw onion through a blender; add 3 oz of liquid honey and 2 1/2 cups of light white wine; take two to four tablespoons a day.

Sage is a tonic that helps the body regain its strength, stimulates appetite, and prevents nocturnal perspiration. Drink a cup after meals and one before going to bed at night. Prepare infusions using 1/2 oz to 2/3 oz of sage per quart of boiled water. To combat night sweats, take between a half and one teaspoon of tincture, mixed with a little water. To prepare the tincture, fill a container with leaves (tightly packed) and cover with twice their volume of 40-proof alcohol; let stand for 15 days.

Thyme is a diuretic and antiseptic that also stimulates perspiration to effectively eliminate toxins. Use 1 oz of thyme per quart of boiled water to prepare infusions and drink three or four cups a day.

Violet is a laxative and diuretic that helps clear the lungs, stimulates expectoration, and reduces fever. The plant is recommended for the treatment of all eruptive and inflammatory disorders.

❧ Memory Loss

What did I do with my keys? Where's my wallet? My gloves? My cell phone? My head?

Plants can't think for you, of course, or remove all your distractions. But they can help keep your mental functions sharp. Practicing meditation and some form of relaxation is also recommended, as the underlying cause of memory loss often turns out to be related to stress or anxiety.

Plant Power

Make sure you're getting enough Vitamins B1, B3, and B6, either in your diet or in supplement form. Then, try some of these remedies to bring back some memories.

Angelica is a general stimulant that balances the nervous system. Infuse 1/3 oz of angelica root in a quart of boiled water for half an hour; drink a cup after meals.

Coriander acts as a stimulant for the mind and body, has a mildly euphoric effect, and improves memory. Infuse two teaspoons of seeds in a cup of water for 10 minutes. Or take half a teaspoon of powdered coriander at a time.

Ginseng generally improves mental functions and combats memory loss. To prepare infusions, use a pinch of ginseng root per cup of boiled water and let stand for 10 minutes. You can also take one vial of liquid ginseng extract per day (not more than 10 days in a row).

Gotu-kola infusions help prevent memory loss. Use a pinch per cup of boiled water and let stand for 10 minutes. If you take gotu-kola liquid extract, stop after 10 days and resume the treatment after waiting 10 days.

Lemon balm (also known as melissa) can be used to treat memory loss related to nervous problems. Use 1/2 oz to 2/3 oz per quart of water to prepare infusions and drink three or four cups a day.

Rosemary is a stimulant that works well for people who are overworked or suffering from fatigue. Soak 2 oz in a quart of good quality wine and drink a glass or two a day.

❧ Menopause Problems

Physiologically speaking, menopause simply signals the reduction (premenopause) and eventual end of menstruation. But the actual experience differs tremendously from woman to woman. For some, there is hardly any change in the way they feel; while for others, a variety of problems crop up: irregular menstruation, hot flashes, high blood pressure, sudden growth of body hair, sexual problems, anxiety, irritability, depression, and even psychosis.

Of course not all women experience these problems, and in most cases the problems they do develop are temporary. Unless you suffer from persistent hot flashes, significant blood loss outside of menstrual periods, or menstruation that lasts for months at a time, there is no need for medical treatment. However, it is a good idea to see a gynecologist more regularly than you might have done in the past.

Plant Power

Exercise and frequent walks outdoors will improve your general state of health during menopause, especially if you remember to do some deep

WHAT TO DO FOR AMENORRHEA

Amenorrhea (interrupted or insufficient menstruation) can happen for many reasons, including excessively strict dieting, obesity, or psychological trauma. Royal jelly and Vitamins A, B1, B3, C, D, and E are all helpful in regulating menstrual flow. So are these common herbs:

- **Angelica** is an effective treatment for insufficient or painful menstruation. Prepare infusions using 1/2 oz to 1 oz of roots or young stems, or 10 to 15 grams of seeds per quart of water.
- **Chamomile** is recommended for cases of painful or irregular menstruation. Use 1 oz to 2 oz of plant per quart of water to prepare infusions and drink a cup an hour before going to bed at night. You can also combine chamomile and sage.
- **Tarragon** facilitates menstruation. Prepare infusions using a tablespoon of plant per cup of boiled water.
- **Lemon balm** regulates menstrual flow and is recommended for cases of amenorrhea. Use 1 oz to 2 oz of flower tops per quart of water to prepare infusions and drink three or four cups a day.
- **Parsley** helps restore normal menstrual flow. Boil 2 oz of parsley roots in a quart of water for 10 minutes; drink three cups a day during the three days preceding your scheduled period and during the first three days of your period.
- **Sage** is a general stimulant that helps restore normal menstrual flow in cases of irregular or insufficient menstruation. Prepare infusions using 2/3 oz of plant per quart of boiled water.

breathing. Avoid sources of fatigue or stress, make sure you get enough sleep, and cut down on your intake of tea, coffee, and alcohol. Then try adding some of these plant remedies to your daily routine.

Yarrow helps regulate menstruation and alleviates anxiety during menopause. Prepare sitz baths by soaking 3 oz of yarrow in a quart of water overnight; in the morning bring to a boil and add to your bath water.

Hawthorn helps lower blood pressure, regulate cardiac activity, and calm the nervous system. This plant is especially recommended for palpitations, hot flashes, insomnia, irritability, or ringing in the ears. To prepare infusions use 1/2 oz to 2/3 oz of leaves per quart of water, and drink two or three cups a day. To combat vaginal dryness, add 1/3 oz each of hawthorn flowers, mistletoe, and sage to a quart of cold water; boil for five minutes, then remove from heat and let stand for 10 minutes; cool until lukewarm and use the liquid for vaginal douches before going to bed at night.

Cypress is another plant that lessens symptoms associated with menopause. Boil 1 oz of freshly crushed nuts in a quart of water for 15 minutes; drink two or three cups a day.

Mistletoe helps alleviate various menopausal symptoms including hot flashes, palpitations, irregular heartbeat, anxiety, and shortness of breath. Soak a teaspoon of mistletoe in a cup of water overnight; in the morning, heat in a double boiler (don't boil), filter, and drink one or two cups a day.

Mint is a mild sedative (unless taken in large doses) that alleviates anxiety and nervousness. It also acts as an antispasmodic. Use 1 oz of leaves and flower tops per quart of water to prepare infusions, and drink two or three cups a day.

Sage stimulates menstrual flow and is recommended for menstrual problems both during puberty and menopause. It also combats fatigue and depression, low blood pressure, and several nervous problems. Taken before bed, it prevents night sweats. Use 2/3 oz per quart of water to prepare infusions, and drink three cups a day, after meals.

✎ Mouth Sores

The extremely painful mouth sores known as aphthous ulcers or canker sores can come from many causes, including thrush (a fungal disease most often contracted by children), stress, trauma, or irritants, such as acidic foods. Despite their unsightly appearance, aphthous ulcers on the tongue, gums, palate, and throat are not difficult to treat. However, if lesions cover a large part of the mouth and are accompanied by bleeding gums and fever, do not hesitate to consult a doctor.

Plant Power

Avoid pork, spicy foods, acidic foods, fats, canned goods, strong alcohol, and other foods that tend to irritate the digestive system. Eat two tablespoons of raw chopped cabbage and one teaspoon of wheat germ per day.

ARE FEVER BLISTERS AND CANKER SORES THE SAME?

Although both occur in or around the mouth and both can be very painful, fever blisters and canker sores are quite different from each other. Here's how:

- Fever blisters are caused by a virus (herpes simplex), while canker sores are usually caused by some local irritant.
- Fever blisters are contagious, while canker sores are not.
- Fever blisters often cause pain even before the actual blister appears, while canker sores are painful onlywhen they ulcerate.

Both last up to 10 days, and unfortunately, there's no actual cure for either, although there are remedies that can speed recovery and reduce pain.

If any sore in the mouth doesn't go away in two weeks, it's important to have your doctor or dentist take a look at it.

Also, try to rest for awhile after your midday meal, and give some of these plant remedies a try.

Agrimony infusions make a good mouthwash: Infuse 2 oz of flowers in a quart of boiled water for one hour; cool, filter, and gargle four times a day.

Burdock, because of its antiseptic properties, makes an effective remedy for all types of skin problems. Drinking three or four cups a day of burdock infusion (1 oz to 2 oz of fresh leaves per quart of boiled water) is a good way to flush toxins out of your organism.

Chamomile decoctions (use Anthemis nobilis chamomile for this disorder) can be very helpful. Add 1 oz of dried flowers to a quart of boiling water, remove from heat, cover, and let stand for about 20 minutes. Drink two or three cups a day.

Mallow extractions, used as a mouthwash, soothe irritation and reduce inflammation. Add 1 oz of mallow root to a quart of water and boil for 15 minutes. Sweeten with a little honey, and drink as many cups as you like during the course of the day.

Walnut is useful because of its antibiotic properties. Boil 1/3 oz of leaves in half a quart of water for 20 minutes; cool to room temperature, and use as a gargle three times a day.

Nettle makes an effective remedy for many types of skin problems, notably because of its antiseptic properties. Use nettle decoctions as a gargle: Boil 2 oz of nettle leaves in a quart of water until a third of the water has evaporated; filter, cool, and gargle three times a day.

Blackberry combats inflammation and accelerates healing of lesions. Use decoctions: Boil 2 oz of leaves in a quart of water for 10 minutes, remove from heat and let stand for 10 minutes. Drink four cups a day, sweetened with a little honey.

Sage is very effective for accelerating the healing of sores. Gargle with sage decoctions four times a day: Simmer 4 oz of leaves in a quart of water for 20 minutes, filter, and cool to room temperature.

Coltsfoot can be used in a lotion that you apply directly to apthis ulcers: Mix 6 drops of essential coltsfoot oil and 3 drops of myrrh tincture with a teaspoon of honey. Apply the lotion regularly for a week to 10 days. *Do not swallow the lotion. Essential oils are extremely concentrated and can be toxic.*

A combination of a number of plants mentioned above can be used to prepare a mouthwash. Mix 2 oz of mallow flowers with 2 oz of blackberry leaves and 3 oz of walnut leaves. Add 2 oz of the mixture to a quart of boiled water and infuse for 20 minutes. Filter, then add about 2 grams of sodium borate. Cool to room temperature and use as a mouthwash four times a day.

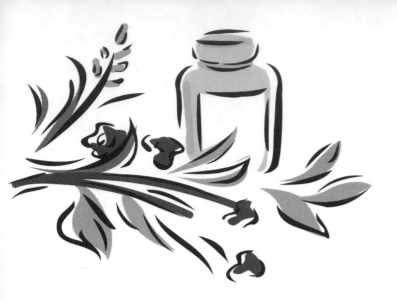

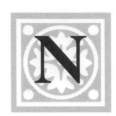

〜 Nail Care

Like your hair, your nails reflect your state of health. Symptoms like white spots, dry brittle nails, or fissured nails can each be the sign of a health problem, such as a vitamin or mineral deficiency, malnutrition, a liver problem, or even angina. Nails that turn black, one after the other, are an indication of gangrene, diabetes, or inflammation of an artery. Some cosmetic products, notably acetone-based polish removers, can also damage nails.

General Care

Wear rubber gloves to do household cleaning, especially if you use chemical detergents or solvents. Women should not keep their nails painted all the time, especially in winter, in order to improve their resistance to cold. A good way to keep nails healthy is to spread a thin layer of pure olive oil on them from time to time.

For healthy toenails, always wear comfortable shoes, and always cut your nails squarely. A rounded shape or tight shoes can cause ingrown toenails.

Plant Power

Absorbing lots of calcium and eating lots of fresh fruit and vegetables is a good way to keep your nails—and the rest of your body—healthy. Vitamins

HOW TO HAVE THE FINGERNAILS YOU'VE ALWAYS WANTED

Having healthy, natural, beautiful nails is easy, if you know how. It's simply a matter of regular, common-sense care. Here's what to do.

Moisturize. Always use a cream or lotion after washing your hands, as soap will tend to dry out your nails and make them crack or chip.

File from corner to middle. Using an emery board or file, shape the nail from the corners inward. And move the file in one direction only. Going back and forth will cause ridges and splitting.

Leave the cuticle alone. Cosmetics counters are full of little gadgets designed to push your cuticles back, but your cuticles are where they are for a reason. They prevent germs and fungus from getting under the skin at the base of the nail. So let them be.

Soak before cleaning. Let your hands sit in warm, soapy water for a few moments before cleaning your nails. Then use an orangewood stick, rather than a metal nail cleaner, to remove dirt from under the nail. The stick is gentler.

D and G are especially important for your nails, so make sure you get enough. These plants can also help.

Lemon strengthens nails: Rub slices of fresh lemon on them once a week.

Malva helps cure nail infections. Soak 2/3 oz of the plant in two quarts of water for a couple of hours; warm slightly and use the liquid for a 20-minute foot or hand bath (the same infusion can be used two or three times).

Onion helps heal brittle or broken nails. Simply cut an onion in half and rub on your nails. You can also use onion juice as a local application. Expect to wait a couple of weeks before seeing results.

Olive helps alleviate pain caused by ingrown nails. Infuse 6 oz to 7 oz of olive leaves in half a quart of boiled water for 15 minutes; filter and use as compresses. Olive oil strengthens nails; once a week, heat a little olive oil in a double boiler and dip your fingers right up to the first knuckle.

Horsetail helps strengthen nails—use it as an internal application, along with lemon and olive oil as external applications. Soak 1 1/2 oz of the plant in a quart of water for three hours; bring to a boil, then simmer for half an hour; remove from heat and let stand for 15 minutes; drink three cups a day, between meals, 15 days per month.

❧ Nervousness

In many cases, being chronically nervous can produce harmful side effects, like insomnia or difficult digestion. Nervousness is also a source of stress, which in turn can develop into more serious disorders like high blood pressure and even cancer.

In most cases it's possible to control nervousness, and sometimes an attack of nerves will even subside on its own. In some cases, however, seeking the help of a qualified health professional, and a period of rest, may be necessary.

Plant Power

Brewer's yeast strengthens the nervous system and helps combat anxiety because of its high Vitamin B content. But you should also try some of the plants listed below. Many have a calming, soothing effect on the nervous system, although you may have to try a few before you find the one that suits you best.

Chamomile is well known for its calming effect and is often prescribed to soothe less severe cases of nervous agitation. Prepare infusions using 1 oz per quart of boiling water and let stand for five minutes. Drink a cup a half hour before meals or an hour after meals.

Lavender has a soothing effect on frayed, sensitive nerves. To prepare infusions use 2/3 oz to 1 oz of flowers per quart of boiling water, and let stand for 10 minutes.

Wild thyme is recommended for cases of depression and over-excitation. You can prepare a soothing wild thyme bath: Soak 8 oz of the plant in a bucket containing about six quarts of water overnight; heat and add to your bath water. Stay in the bath for about 20 minutes, keeping your heart above the surface. When you come out of the bath, wrap yourself in a large towel or bathrobe to stimulate perspiration, and rest for about half an hour.

Valerian is a sedative that can be very effective for treating nervous problems, agitation, palpitations, or feelings of aggression. It can also be used to calm nervous children. It is important, however, to respect the recommended dosage, because taking too much valerian will produce the opposite effect (i.e., it will make you even more nervous). To prepare a valerian tincture, soak 1-1/2 oz of dried, ground roots in a cup of 60-proof alcohol for two days, stirring occasionally. Take 10 to 15 drops at a time, three times a day.

Mistletoe makes an effective remedy for soothing frayed nerves. Boil 1 oz of the plant in a quart of water for 10 minutes; sweeten with honey, and add a pinch of aniseed to taste; drink three or four cups a day.

Hawthorn is an antispasmodic that has a sedative effect on nervous disorders (anxiety, insomnia, etc.). This plant is recommended for persons who are overworked, highly emotional, or irritable, or who suffer from nervous spasms. Infuse 1/2 oz to 2/3 oz of flowers in a quart of water for 10 minutes; drink two to four cups a day, for a maximum of 2/3 oz on consecutive days.

Black hemp nettle calms frayed nerves, improves sleep, and alleviates various symptoms, including anxiety, dizziness, hot flashes, and palpitations. To prepare your own tincture, soak a heaping cup of the plant in two cups of

MEDITATE YOUR NERVES AWAY

Meditation is a great way to relax, and relaxation is one of the best methods for thwarting a nervous attack. Here's how to get started.

First, find a comfortable, softly lit spot where you're not likely to be disturbed by people or distracted by noise. Then, sit comfortably on a chair. Keep your feet on the floor and your back straight. It may help to sit on the edge of the chair, rather than leaning against the back. Lay one hand on top of each leg—palm up or palm down makes no difference.

Now, either close your eyes or let them remain slightly open while focusing on a spot on the floor in front of you. Begin to breathe deeply, and exhale very slowly. After you've done this a few times, try to become aware of how each part of your body feels. If you find tension anywhere, allow those muscles to relax. If any thoughts or distractions try to get your attention, don't fight them. Just be aware of them and let them go on their own.

Meditating like this for just a few minutes each day will go a long way toward making your nervous attacks things of the past.

eau-de-vie or brandy for 15 days; filter and store in a sealed container. Dosage: three or four teaspoons per day.

Hops have a calming, tranquilizing effect. An effective treatment for insomnia, hops are also anaphrodisiac (i.e., they inhibit sexual desire). Prepare infusions using 1/2 oz to 1 oz of cones per quart of water, and drink three or four cups a day.

Marjoram is an antispasmodic recommended for difficult digestion related to nervous problems, anxiety, insomnia, facial spasms, etc. Infuse 1 oz to 2 oz of leaves in a quart of boiled water for 10 minutes, and drink one or two cups a day.

Lemon balm (melissa) is a sedative, antispasmodic, and stimulant that helps calm nervous, irritable, agitated, or depressed persons. It acts as both a sedative and a natural tonic. Use 2/3 oz of flower tops per quart of water to prepare infusions and drink three or four cups a day. You can also combine lemon balm and citronella (1/2 oz of each in a cup of boiling water), adding a zest of lemon and some honey. Drink a cup before going to bed at night.

Orange is a mild sedative that calms the nervous system and combats insomnia. It is recommended for persons suffering from anxiety, spasms, nervous palpitations, or general agitation and also helps combat head and stomach aches. Prepare infusions using 1/2 oz per quart of water.

Thyme in your bath water will calm agitation (recommended for both children and adults). Soak 6 oz of thyme in six to eight quarts of water overnight. Heat, and add to your bath water.

Linden has a sedative, relaxing effect. Use it to calm mental agitation and combat insomnia, either alone as an infusion or mixed with hawthorn.

Speedwell is recommended for cases of nervousness related to intellectual exhaustion and helps improve memory functions. Drink a cup of infusion before going to bed at night.

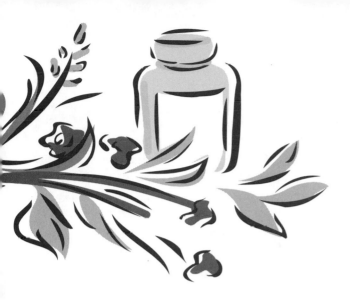

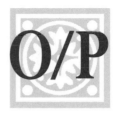

≈ Pain

Pain, to quote an old saw, is nature's way of telling you that something's wrong. If it's external pain, you probably know what caused it—a stubbed toe or a toothache. But pain on the inside is a different story. It might be something as trivial as a little gas or as serious as a stomach ulcer, as passing as a tension headache or as catastrophic as an impending stroke. That's why it's important to know the cause. If you have a pain and you don't know what's causing it, see a health professional.

Plant Power

Whatever the cause of your pain, there's no reason why you

NEW CURE FOR PAIN?

Could the sap of a common South American tree be a new miracle cure for pain? Some researchers think so.

The sap, called Sangre de Grado, has been used for centuries by Indian tribes along the Amazon River basin as an herbal medicine to treat wounds and relieve pain. Recent research shows these tribes were onto something.

Laboratory tests show not only that Sangre de Grado relieves pain, but that it also blocks inflammation—and it does it both internally and externally. Whether your pain is from a wound on the skin or from an infection in your stomach, the sap still works!

One field study in Louisiana showed that outdoor workers who used the sap to treat insect bites and stings got potent pain relief within 90 seconds!

Although the product isn't available for human consumption yet in the United States, researchers hope that the day when it will be isn't far off.

NEURALGIA

Neuralgia is the medical term for nerve pain. A pins-and-needles sensation and loss of sensitivity surrounding the affected nerve also come with the condition.

What to do about it? Vitamin B1 (thiamin) helps prevent neuralgia by nourishing the nerves, but if you're already coping with the condition, try rubbing some chamomile oil over the affected area. It's easy to make. Soak 3 oz of German chamomile in a quart of warm oil for two hours; filter and massage it into the skin.

For facial neuralgia, try this: 1/3 oz each of chamomile, mullein, yarrow, and thyme; place them all in a sachet and apply directly to the affected area.

Cloves help alleviate dental neuralgic pain: Simply place a clove on the painful tooth while waiting to see your dentist.

should have to tolerate it without relief. Here is nature's best cure for soothing your discomfort.

Poplar has a sedative effect, and can help fight pain caused by rheumatism, gout, abscesses, ulcers, and many other causes, all without the side effects of most over-the-counter pain relievers. Prepare decoctions using 1 oz of buds per quart of water and drink four or five cups during the course of the day.

∽ Perspiration (Excessive)

Perspiration, far from being harmful, is essential for health. It helps to keep your body from becoming overheated, and it flushes toxins from your system.

However, when you sweat so much that it interferes with your daily activities or when your sweat gives off an unpleasant odor, it's time to do something about it.

General Care

One way to combat excessive perspiration of the feet is to take alternating hot and cold foot baths every day. If foot odor is a problem, make sure to keep your feet clean, change your socks frequently, and powder your feet and shoes with talc.

As for the rest of the body, it's best to wear cotton instead of wool or synthetic clothing, because cotton is a breathing fiber that absorbs perspiration and keeps you from becoming overheated. You can also try adding some sage to your bath water.

Plant Power

Your diet has a direct effect on how much you perspire. If perspiration is a problem, adopt a diet that resembles the hypotoxic diet. Eat frugally, reduce your intake of fats, and drink less coffee, beer, etc. Then try some of these plant remedies.

Birch is a diuretic that stimulates elimination of waste through urine. Infuse 1 oz of leaves in a quart of water for 10 minutes, add a pinch of bicarbonate of soda, and drink two cups a day. You can also combine birch and sage.

Sage is recommended for cases of excessive perspiration, unless you suffer from bladder or intestinal inflammation. Applied externally, it helps prevent nocturnal perspiration and neutralizes foot and body odors: Infuse 2 oz in two quarts of water for 10 minutes, and apply to the feet, under the arms, etc. You can also buy sage essence in most pharmacies and herbal or health food stores: Simply add a few drops to your bath water. For internal use, drink a cup of sage tea before going to bed at night: Infuse 1 oz of leaves in a quart of water for 15 minutes.

✒ Phlebitis

Phlebitis is the medical term for inflammation of a vein in the legs caused by the formation of a blood clot, and it can be dangerous. If the vein becomes completely blocked, the condition is known as thrombophlebitis. The condition should be closely monitored by a doctor, because there is always a danger of the clot moving through the bloodstream and into the lungs—a situation that is life threatening.

Symptoms include feet and calves becoming sensitive to touch and, in some cases, painful; fever; and accelerated pulse.

LEG PROBLEMS

Phlebitis isn't the only problem your legs can give you. Cramps and stiffness can also be annoying, if not downright debilitating. Fortunately, there are ways of preventing these conditions.

If your work forces you to remain standing for long periods of time, stretch out on your back with your legs raised above the rest of your body for 10 minutes at the end of each working day. Also try standing on tiptoe a few times when you get up in the morning, and as often as possible during the course of the day. The bicycle exercise is also effective: Lie on your back with your legs in a vertical position in the air and move them round and round as if you were pedaling a bicycle. Continue for 15 minutes, taking a short break every four or five minutes.

One way to alleviate a feeling of heaviness in the legs, as well as swollen feet, is to bathe them in water that has been used to cook potatoes or other vegetables. Afterwards apply hot salt compresses (heat in the oven before wrapping around the feet). Or add some sea salt to bath water containing a hay flower infusion.

People sometimes develop phlebitis after undergoing surgery, giving birth, suffering some kind of physical injury, or having an abortion.

General Care

You should stay in bed while waiting to see a doctor. Gentle massaging of the leg while raising the ankles and pressing them toward the thighs can be helpful (twice a day, morning and evening). Medical treatments include the prescribing of an anticoagulant to dislodge the clot, and physiotherapy on affected limbs.

Plant Power

Diet should be largely vegetarian, consisting mainly of fruit, vegetables, and low-fat dairy products. Plants can be used as a complement to conventional medical treatment.

Garlic can be used to prepare compresses for local application: Prepare a decoction using one whole garlic bulb, 1 oz of coltsfoot, and 1 oz of yarrow per quart of water; soak some gauze or clean cotton in the decoction and apply to affected areas.

Nettle foot baths stimulate circulation: Soak 1 1/2 oz of freshly grated roots and 1 1/2 oz of leaves and stems in two quarts of water overnight; bring to a boil and use to bathe your feet (the bath should be as hot as possible).

Marigold ointment can help cure some cases of phlebitis. Put two heaping cups of fresh flowers, stems, and leaves through a blender; add the ground plant to 1 lb of melted lard (temperature should not be higher than 212 degrees Fahrenheit); remove from heat, filter through cheesecloth or fine cotton, and let stand for a day. Filter again through some fine cotton, and store in clean glass containers. Apply a thick layer of the ointment to affected areas daily.

Coltsfoot works well for external applications. Prepare an ointment with ground leaves, mixed with fresh cream, and apply to inflamed areas.

➥ Pneumonia

Although the term pneumonia can refer to any type of lung infection, whether it's caused by a virus, a fungus, or even a chemical, it's the bacterial variety, pneumococcal pneumonia, that is of the gravest concern for public health. According to the National Institutes of Health, it is the leading cause of serious illness in the world today, and accounts for 40,000 deaths every year in the United States.

Pneumococcal pneumonia generally appears after a bout of flu or some other type of infection. It can appear suddenly, causing a piercing pain in the ribs, high fever, and bacteria-infested phlegm.

Modern antibiotics are generally effective for curing the problem, but elderly persons have to be careful as heart failure is always a possibility.

Plant Power

Consult a doctor as soon as possible in order to obtain a prescription for an appropriate antibiotic. The plants listed below are useful only for complementary treatment.

Angelica is recommended for the treatment of most pulmonary disorders. Combine it with horehound, 1/2 oz each of angelica root and horehound flower tops, infused in a quart of boiled water for about 10 minutes; drink three or four cups a day.

Borage has an anti-inflammatory effect. Boil 1 oz of dried plant in a quart of water for 10 minutes (add the plant to cold water and bring to a boil); drink five or six cups during the course of the day.

Common broom, recommended for the treatment of acute pulmonary disorders, helps respiration, tones the heart, and acts as a diuretic. Use 1 oz to 2 oz of fresh young flowers per quart of water to prepare infusions and drink between two and four cups a day.

Marigold is an antiseptic and anti-inflammatory that promotes flushing of toxins through perspiration. Prepare infusions using 1 oz of flowers per quart of water, or combine it with equal amounts of wild pansy flowers, borage, and common broom; mix well and infuse 1 oz of the mixture in a quart of boiled water for 10 minutes.

DO HERBS HAVE A ROLE IN PREGNANCY?

Because a fetus is so sensitive to substances introduced into its mother's system, we don't recommend taking herbal remedies during pregnancy unless you're under the care of a qualified herbalist.

There are certain plants that you must absolutely avoid. These include absinthe, mountain wormwood, celandine, berberis (also known as barberry), male fern, juniper, mandrake, marjoram, oregano, pennyroyal, rosemary, rue, tansy, thyme, saffron, and blood root.

Rosemary, thyme, sage, marjoram, and parsley present no danger when used as condiments on salads or for cooking. However, pregnant women should not take therapeutic doses of these plants.

Pregnancy

Pregnancy is an especially important and vulnerable time in the lives of a mother and the child she is carrying. That's why mothers should never take any kind of medication, even an over-the-counter product such as aspirin, unless they are absolutely sure it is safe.

X-rays can also be dangerous, especially as a mother approaches the end of her term. Some experts even claim that expecting mothers should not spend too much time in front of the TV set because of the electromagnetic rays the device emits.

Lifestyle

You are making decisions for two people, instead of just for yourself. Smoking while pregnant is not a criminal offense. But if you want to give your child the best possible start in life, why not make an effort to stop these harmful habits, at least while you are carrying your child and breast-feeding (nicotine, for example, makes its way into a mother's milk in a matter of hours).

Drinking is another story. Studies show that even small amounts of alcohol can lead to fetal alcohol syndrome, which can cause a host of problems ranging from lowered IQ to extreme behavior problems, and even death.

Nutrition

Is a mother's diet a determining factor as far as the health of her child is concerned? No one can say for sure. It is certain, however, that nutrition, along with a mother's mental attitude and physical condition, is a crucial aspect of any successful pregnancy.

Eat at regular hours and chew your food well so that it will be assimilated more easily. You don't have to start eating more than usual until about the fifth month or so.

Cut down on coffee and tea, and eat more mineral-rich foods such as cabbage, spinach, carrots, and parsley (preferably raw, either grated or chopped, added to salads). Eat more fruit and vegetables in general. As for meat, opt for roasted or grilled methods of cooking, and avoid fat and greasy sauces. Also reduce your intake of fish (unless it is very fresh), pasta, pastry, and other starchy foods.

Milk and other calcium-rich foods contain important proteins that pregnant women need. A little liver from time to time will help the fetus build up its iron reserves.

Morning Sickness

Nausea and vomiting during pregnancy should not be taken lightly. If morning sickness becomes seriously unpleasant, therapeutic measures should be taken. The fact that morning sickness is often alleviated by chewing on a piece of dry toast indicates that the problem is hypoglycemia. However, before taking any kind of medication or herbal remedy, consult a qualified specialist.

➣ Prostate Problems

The prostate is a uniquely male gland, situated just in front of the rectum and behind the scrotum. It's about the size of a walnut when it's healthy, but it can swell to a larger size due to infection or a common male condition called BPH (benign prostatic hyperplasia), which men often get after the age of 50.

Prostatitis (inflammation of the prostate gland) is characterized by high fever, difficulty urinating, and pain in the genital region.

General Care

Conventional medical treatment relies on antibiotics to cure prostatitis. However, it is also important to determine the underlying cause of the problem to prevent recurrences and to avoid the risk of an abscess forming in the prostate gland or of missing the diagnosis of a tumor.

Daily hot sitz baths before going to bed at night are recommended. Hot rectal enemas (120 degrees Fahrenheit) help alleviate feelings of heaviness and urine retention if the liquid is retained in the rectum for at least half an hour. Also, sleep on your side, and make sure to urinate before going to bed at night and whenever you feel the need during the night.

THE TELLTALE SIGNS OF PROSTATE CANCER

Prostate health is one of those things that men need to be aware of, just as women need to be aware of breast health. And like breast cancer in women, prostate cancer is something men need to watch out for.

Your risk for getting prostate cancer is higher if you're over 50, are black, or have a family history of the disease.

The symptoms of prostate cancer can mimic those of many other conditions that are far less dangerous, so if any of the following signs pertain to you, you'll need to see a urologist for an evaluation:

- Frequent trips to the bathroom, especially at night
- A weak stream when you urinate
- Urgent need to urinate
- Straining to start or finish urinating
- Lower back pain
- Bloody urine

Sometimes, prostate cancer shows no symptoms at all, so if you're over 40, a regular exam—both digital and blood sample—are a must.

Plant Power

A frugal diet is best: Try to adopt a hypotoxic diet, at least until the problem is resolved. Also try some of the plants listed below for relief. A note of caution: You *won't* see saw palmetto, a common herb for the treatment of BPH, listed below. Although saw palmetto does indeed reduce the symptoms of that condition, it can also mask the symptoms of prostate cancer. For that reason, it's not recommended, unless you take it under a doctor's care.

Broom heather increases urine volume, facilitates elimination of waste, has an antiseptic effect on the urinary tract, and alleviates prostate inflammation. Boil 1 oz of flower tops in a quart of water until a third of the water has evaporated. Drink two or three cups a day.

Bearberry is a diuretic, sedative, and disinfectant that can help fight urinary and genital infections. Use decoctions or a concentrated maceration and drink about a cup per day. To prepare decoctions, boil 1 oz of dried leaves in a quart of water until a quarter of the water has evaporated. The maceration is more active: Bring 1 oz of crushed leaves to a boil, then remove from heat and let stand overnight; in the morning stir and filter. *Note: Never use metal containers or utensils to work with this plant.*

Willow is reputed to be an extremely effective remedy for prostate inflammation and other prostate problems. Some experts even claim it can cure cancer of the prostate gland.

Goldenseal is a tonic that helps combat infections. Take 10 to 20 drops of goldenseal extract (available in pharmacies and health food and herbal stores) every hour.

Pellitory-of-the-wall is a depurative (it cleans the blood) and an emollient (it alleviates inflammation). Extract the juice by putting the plant through an extractor and take three to five teaspoons per day. Or drink as much decoction as you like: Add 2 oz of the plant to a quart of cold water, boil for five minutes, then remove from heat and let stand for 10 minutes.

Pine cones have a diuretic and antiseptic effect on the urinary tract. Infuse 1 oz of cones in a quart of water for one hour; sweeten with honey.

ᔥ Psoriasis

Conventional medicine considers psoriasis incurable. Yet homeopathic and plant treatments can produce excellent results. If you are undergoing sulfur, tar, mercury, or X-ray treatments, however, natural remedies are less likely to be effective.

Heredity is one major cause of psoriasis, although psychological factors also play a role, which is why homeopathic doctors often prescribe different remedies for the problem, depending on the character of the patient.

Initial symptoms include well-defined spots of varying dimensions that appear on the skin, especially on the knees, elbows, and back. Dry scaly skin then forms over affected areas. Skin underneath is shiny, red, and very fragile. Itching can be very intense.

General Care

With a little effort in your daily life, you can keep your psoriasis under control. Here's how.

Nix the bad habits. Psoriasis is often linked to alcohol consumption and cigarette smoking. If you suffer from psoriasis and drink or smoke, try to stop as soon as possible.

Add starch. Bathing affected areas in starchy water helps alleviate itching. Add 2 tablespoons of corn starch to your bath water.

Take your vitamins. Make sure you are getting enough Vitamins A, C, and D. These all promote healthy skin.

Try some fat. To relieve discomfort, cover lesions with fine lard every day, or use celandine ointment if psoriasis lesions form crusts (use an extractor to obtain 1/4 oz of fresh celandine juice and mix with 2 oz of fine lard; store in your refrigerator).

Detoxify. In addition to external treatments, take some kind of purgative: buckthorn (1 oz per quart of water, infused for 15 minutes) or elder (2/3 oz of elder juice per day).

Plant Power

Ideally you should adopt a hypotoxic diet for a period of three months. Make unrefined brown rice cooked in salted water along with homemade fruit juices a staple of your diet. Drinking freshly pressed vegetable and fruit juices on a regular basis helps prevent psoriasis. Also take fresh brewer's yeast every day. And use these plant remedies for maximum control.

Burdock can be used internally (boil 2 oz of fresh roots for about 10 minutes) or externally (use 3 oz of fresh roots per quart of water).

Barley is an emollient and diuretic. Soak 1 oz to 2 oz of barley in a quart of water for a few hours, then boil over low heat for 20 minutes; drink three cups a day, before noon.

Wild pansy is a depurative and diuretic that is recommended for a variety of skin problems, including psoriasis. Use the sap (2 oz to 3 oz per day, obtained by putting the fresh plant through an extractor), infusions (1 oz of plant per quart of water), or decoctions (2/3 oz of dried plant per quart of water). You can also mix wild pansy with elm bark and Alpine yarrow: Put a handful of each in an enamel pot and add half a quart of boiling water; let stand overnight, then filter through a fine cloth and sweeten with honey; take 10 to 12 tablespoons a day.

Sage lotions help alleviate itching: Simply bathe affected areas with a sage infusion: 1 oz of flower tops per quart of boiled water.

Violet can be used both internally and externally. Simply crush some fresh leaves and apply directly to affected areas, or boil 1 oz of leaves and flowers in a quart of water for 10 minutes and drink three cups in the morning before breakfast.

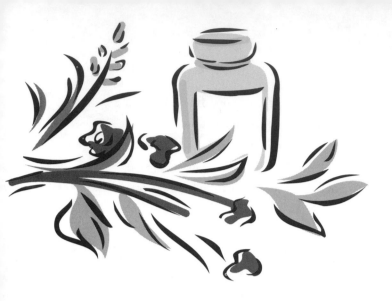

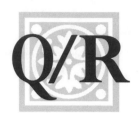

🍂 Rheumatism

In the world of the Hollywood stereotype, an old codger with a charming limp and a lovable but cantankerous attitude complains about his bones whenever the weather changes. But in reality, rheumatism—more properly called rheumatoid arthritis—can be a devastating disease that causes inflammation of the membrane lining the joints. The result can be crippling pain, stiffness, redness, swelling, and damaged and misshapen bone and cartilage. Fortunately, we're not helpless to fight back.

Lifestyle

Hot, dry climates are generally more comfortable for people with rheumatism than are damp, cold, windy climates, so if you live in a northern climate, try to travel south during cold weather. No matter where you live, however, it helps to be able to get out in the warm sun on a fairly regular basis. A minimum of exercise is also necessary, because a sedentary life will only aggravate the condition.

General Care

If you have pain but no inflammation, gentle massage can help prevent muscles from becoming atrophied. Hot air and warm infrared light can help soothe pain in some cases. Hot baths with some algae added, or hot showers, preferably with a massaging shower head, can also alleviate joint pain.

Hot wax treatments can cure rheumatic ankylosis (stiffening of the joint) of the wrists in its early stages. All you have to do is plunge affected wrists into some hot liquid wax and allow the heat and fat contained in the wax to take effect.

MIXING IT UP TO FIGHT RHEUMATISM

This herbal mixture is effective for the treatment of rheumatism. Chop and mix these plants: 15 grams each of buckthorn, burdock, birch, and wild pansy; 2/3 oz each of chamomile, horsetail, and parsley; and 1 oz of juniper berries. Use three teaspoons per cup to prepare infusions; drink a cup in the morning before breakfast and one after each meal for a period of two to three weeks.

Nutrition

Adopt a hypotoxic diet, or at least limit your meat intake as much as possible (two or three meat dishes a week is sufficient). Although brewer's yeast is recommended for a wide variety of health problems, rheumatic sufferers should avoid this supplement. Ideally, you should fast for a day or two a few times a year.

Eat more asparagus, artichoke, tomato, cabbage, chervil, lettuce, pineapple, grapes, bananas, and apples. Celery and potatoes, ingested in large amounts, help prevent rheumatism.

Plant Power

The plants mentioned below can be very helpful for the treatment of rheumatism and are much better than chemical sedatives or analgesics. Many are diuretics, which help eliminate waste through urination.

Garlic produces a sensation of heat that helps reduce rheumatic discomfort. Apply crushed cloves, covered with gauze to hold in place, directly to affected areas for 10 minutes.

Wild garlic is a depurative that is recommended for the treatment of rheumatism. Prepare your own garlic liqueur: Fill a container with fresh leaves and cover with 40-proof alcohol; seal the container and let stand in direct sunlight or near some other heat source for two weeks; take 10 to 15 drops, mixed with a little water, four times a day.

Burdock is a diuretic and depurative that is frequently prescribed for cases of arthritis and rheumatism. Boil 2 oz of fresh roots in a quart of water for 10 minutes and drink three cups a day. If you can't find fresh roots, use stabilized burdock extract, available at pharmacies and health food and herbal stores.

Birch is a diuretic that helps combat rheumatic symptoms. Use 1/2 oz to 1 1/2 oz of young leaves per quart of water to prepare infusions, and drink between three and five cups a day. Or drink birch sap, which you can obtain by piercing the trunk of a birch tree.

Chamomile helps alleviate rheumatic pain. Gently massage painful joints with chamomile oil: Add 2 oz of dried flowers to half a quart of olive oil, and heat for three hours over a double boiler; filter and add 1/3 oz of camphor.

Cabbage leaf compresses alleviate rheumatic pain. Wash a couple of leaves and flatten them with a rolling pin, then apply directly to affected joints, using strips of gauze to hold them in place. Change compresses twice a day.

Watercress is a diuretic and depurative. Drink 3 oz to 5 oz of fresh juice per day, obtained by putting the plant through an extractor, or grinding with a mortar and pestle.

Fennel is another diuretic plant. Boil 1 oz of roots in a quart of water for five minutes, then remove from heat and let stand for 10 minutes. Or infuse 1/2 oz to 1 oz of seeds in a quart of water. Drink three or four cups a day.

Devil's claw (harpagophytum) is reputed to combat arthritis and rheumatism. Soak a tablespoon in half a quart of cold water overnight; next day boil for three minutes, then remove from heat and infuse for 10 minutes; filter and add enough mineral water to make one quart; sweeten with honey to mask the bitter taste. Drink half a quart a day for 10 days, stop for 10 days, then repeat the cycle.

Corn can be used as an internal or external treatment to combat rheumatism. For internal applications, boil 1 oz of dried stalks in a quart of water for 20 minutes, and drink two cups a day. For local applications, prepare some thick corn (or millet) cereal and apply as hot as possible.

St. John's wort oil soothes rheumatic pain. Fill a container with fresh leaves (don't pack them too tightly) and cover with extra virgin olive oil; seal the container and place in direct sunlight or near some other heat source for a few days; when the oil has taken on a characteristic red color, filter through a fine cloth and apply to painful joints.

Nettle is a diuretic and depurative that cleans out your organism and is especially recommended during acute rheumatic phases. Boil 1 oz of roots in a quart of water for 10 minutes and drink three or four cups a day. You can also take nettle baths: Soak 7 oz of nettle in a couple of quarts of water overnight; next day heat the mixture and add it to your bath water; stay in the bath for 20 minutes, with your heart above water level; after the bath don't towel dry—instead wrap yourself in a large towel or bathrobe and stretch out for an hour or so.

Wild pansy is a diuretic, depurative, and mild laxative. Boil 1 oz of fresh plant in a quart of water for a few minutes and drink two or three cups a day, one before breakfast in the morning.

Parsley is a diuretic and depurative that is recommended for cases of chronic rheumatism. Take a teaspoon of fresh parsley juice every morning when you wake up (put some fresh parsley through a juice extractor, or use a mortar and pestle).

Dandelion is a depurative that promotes secretions of bile. Boil 2 oz of dandelion leaves in a quart of water for a few minutes and drink three to six cups a day.

Primrose (also called cowslip) helps alleviate joint pain. Boil 2 oz to 2 1/2 oz in a quart of water, then soak strips of cloth in the decoction and apply as compresses to affected areas.

Wild radish is a diuretic when used internally. Boil 1/3 oz of fresh roots in a quart of water for 10 minutes and take a teaspoon after meals. Used externally, the plant alleviates rheumatic pain. Apply poultices of grated radish to affected joints for 15 minutes, wrapped in gauze. Or put the roots through a blender and add a little oil.

Queen of the meadow is a diuretic that helps eliminate uric acid and chloride and is one of the most effective plants for combating rheumatic symptoms. Use 1 oz of flower tops (fresh if possible) per quart of water to prepare infusions and drink two to four cups a day. Note: Make sure not to boil this plant—water poured over the flower tops should not exceed 190 degrees Fahrenheit.

Rosemary can be applied externally to help alleviate and soothe pain. Use 1 1/2 oz of plant per quart of water to prepare infusions, then dip strips of cloth in the liquid and apply as compresses to affected joints.

Sage also helps alleviate rheumatic pain. Simply add a handful of the plant to your bath water.

Elder is a diuretic and depurative that stimulates perspiration. Boil 1 1/2 oz to 2 oz of leaves and bark (the second layer of bark is best) in a quart of water until half the water has evaporated and drink two or three cups a day.

Thyme decoctions (1 oz to 1 1/2 oz per quart of water) or thyme oil are both recommended for external applications. To prepare your own oil, fill a container with leaves and flowers, then cover with extra virgin olive oil and let stand in direct sunlight or near some other heat source for two weeks. (Essential oil of thyme is available in most pharmacies and health food and herbal stores.)

Verbena infusions have a diuretic effect and help combat rheumatic symptoms. Use 1 oz of leaves or flowers per quart of water and drink two or three cups a day.

❧ Ringing in the Ears

If it occurs only once in awhile, ringing in the ears (tinnitus) is a minor problem. But when it occurs with any regularity, it can be a major distraction.

Many things can cause that irritating, high-pitched sound, including circulation problems and high blood pressure. It can also be triggered by an ear disorder, in which case an ear, nose, and throat specialist should be consulted.

Plant Power

Hawthorn regulates cardiac and nervous functions and can be effective for the treatment of recurring tinnitus. Prepare infusions using 1/3 oz of flower tops per quart of boiling water and let stand for 15 minutes. Remember that hawthorn can be toxic when taken in very large doses, although there is no danger when the plant is used as an infusion.

Black horehound (also known as black hemp nettle) has a calming affect, and can calm anxiety and tension related to psychological stress. Because of the plant's bitter taste, use it in tincture form: Chop up a sufficient quantity of fresh plant and soak in an equal amount of 95-proof alcohol for two weeks; filter and take 25 to 30 drops morning and night.

Rosacea

People used to think that a bright red nose or crimson cheeks were a sure sign of alcoholism. Today we know better. The red skin blotches characteristic of rosacea are the result of dilating blood vessels just beneath the surface of the skin. It usually happens to people in their 30s or 40s, most often those with light complexions who blush or flush easily. The condition may be aggravated, but not caused, by alcohol abuse. Hot drinks, spicy foods, stress, sunlight, and extreme heat or cold can also start a flare-up. As the condition progresses, hard, little pimple-like nodules can appear on the

---

SKIN CARE FOR ROSACEA

The way you wash and care for your facial skin can make a big difference in your appearance if you have rosacea. Here are some do's and don'ts.

Go mild. Use cream-based, mild soaps when you wash. Avoid anything that has alcohol, acetone, or astringents in it.

Moisturize. Always use a topical moisturizer after you wash or after you apply medication (wait for the medication to dry first).

Use sun sense. Stay out of the sun as much as you can, and if you must expose yourself to it, wear a sunscreen of SPF 15 or higher.

Take care not to clog. Use products that are designed not to clog your pores. That means look for the word *noncomedogenic* on the package.

skin, and then the spidery lines of blood vessels. In advanced stages, especially in men, little knots may grow on the nose, which will give it a bulbous appearance.

Plant Power

Although there is no known cure for rosacea, we can control it with medication, either applied topically or taken by mouth. We can also help to keep the skin healthy looking by using the plants listed below.

Lily can be infused to make lily water, which you should apply regularly to affected areas: 3 oz of flowers per half quart of boiling water; remove from heat and let stand for three hours.

Common lettuce soothes and decongests the skin and can be an effective treatment for rosacea. Wash some leaves well, then simmer for two hours. Apply when still warm and leave in place for about half an hour.

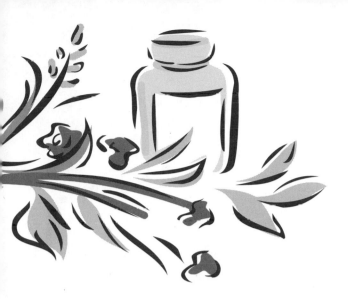

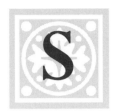

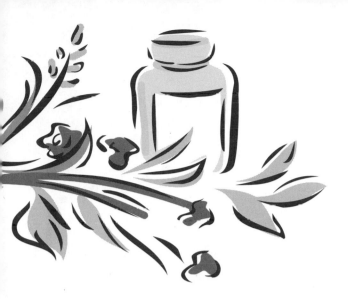 Sciatica

Sciatica is that pain that starts in your lower back or butt and shoots down your thighs and calves to your feet. It's caused by compression of the sciatic nerve, which in turn is caused by the displacement of a disc between the lumbar vertebrae. You probably got it by straining or injuring your lower back. And it's no fun. So what do you do about it?

General Care

Rest is essential—attempting to ignore the pain and carry on with your daily routine will only aggravate the problem. Move the affected limb regularly to prevent stiffening or deformation.

A doctor will usually prescribe a pain killer and an anti-inflammatory medication. A chiropractor or osteopath can sometimes remedy the situation rapidly by realigning the lumbar vertebrae.

Plant Power

Plants can't put vertebrae back into place, of course, but they can help you to feel more comfortable, and they can reduce inflammation. Here are some to try.

White bryony can be applied externally to reduce pain. Prepare poultices using freshly grated pulp. You can also mix the pulp or sap with some soft bread.

Cabbage poultices are also effective: Place a couple of cabbage leaves between two pieces of cloth and heat with an iron, then apply directly to the painful area. Change the poultice twice a day.

St. John's wort oil works well when rubbed on affected areas. Fill a container with fresh leaves (don't pack too tightly) and cover with pure virgin olive oil; seal the container and let stand in direct sunlight or near some other heat source; when the mixture turns red, filter through a fine cloth.

Queen of the meadow is a diuretic, antispasmodic, and anti-inflammatory plant that helps alleviate sciatic pain. Use 1 oz of flower tops (fresh if possible) per quart of water to prepare infusions, making sure not to boil the plant (water should not be hotter than 190 degrees Fahrenheit); drink two to four cups a day.

Nettle helps cure some cases of sciatica. Rub affected areas with fresh nettle and take nettle baths: Soak 7 oz of the plant in a couple of quarts of water overnight; next morning heat and add to your bath water; stay in the bath for 20 minutes, keeping your heart above water level. After the bath, wrap yourself in a warm bathrobe or large towel, without rubbing yourself dry, and stretch out for an hour.

Linden is an antispasmodic and mild sedative that helps alleviate sciatic pain. Combine 1/3 oz of linden with a pinch each of red poppy flowers, hops, and passion flower; infuse the mixture in a quart of water for about 10 minutes and drink a cup in the evening to help you sleep.

❧ Senility

As we get older and the changes aging brings to us seem to creep into every corner of our lives, it's easy to become anxious, if not downright frightened. We forget where we put our keys or an old friend's name slips our mind, and we immediately feel as if we're on the verge of losing our thinking faculties altogether. We imagine becoming helpless and feeble, unable to get to the bathroom without the help of a nurse.

We should stop scaring ourselves that way. The fact is, with a little common sense and good health habits, we can greatly reduce our chance of becoming senile in our later years.

General Care

There arc many therapies designed to restore the vigor of youth: hormone treatments, placenta-based serums, cellular injections, procaine injections, etc. These strategies provide temporary relief at best. They can't make up for a lifetime of smoking, drinking, lack of exercise, or eating bad foods.

The best way to retard the aging process and prevent senility from setting in is to stay healthy in spirit, mind, and body, and eat the right kinds of food.

Plant Power

Foods that are rich in iodine have a beneficial effect on us as we age. Some iodine-rich foods include green leafy vegetables, watercress, asparagus, carrots, cod liver oil, and fish in general. You can also add some of these youth-enhancing remedies to your daily diet.

Blueberry wine is a delicious and effective anti-aging remedy: Pour a quart of white wine over 2 oz of blueberry leaves; let stand for a couple of days, then filter through a fine cloth; drink two glasses a day. You can also mix blueberry with queen of the meadow, ash, and mint (1/2 oz of each); infuse for 10 minutes in a quart of boiled water, and drink five or six cups during the course of the day.

Nasturtium is rich in sulfur essences, phosphoric acid, and vitamin C, all of which help combat senility. It is also considered an aphrodisiac. Add it to salads or drink decoctions: Use 1 oz of plant per quart of boiling water. Preparing a nasturtium liqueur allows you to keep the remedy handy all year long: Tightly fill a container with fresh leaves and cover with an equal volume of eau-de-vie or brandy; let stand for 15 days, then store in a sealed container; take a teaspoon three times a day.

Blackcurrant is a diuretic and depurative (it cleans the blood) that also combats rheumatism. The berries are rich in vitamin C and taste delicious. Soak two handfuls of leaves in a quart of white or red wine; filter and store in a cool place.

➤ Shingles

Shingles is a skin disease caused by a virus that resembles the chickenpox virus. It generally affects middle-aged and elderly persons. Symptoms include burning pain that lasts for a few days, followed by eruptions that turn red and develop small white blisters. Crusts disappear leaving white scars.

Curing shingles can be difficult—treatments take at least a few weeks, often longer for elderly people. Consulting a doctor is essential. Antibiotics are almost always prescribed to prevent secondary infections, but homeopathic doctors can cure the condition without resorting to antibiotic medications.

General Care

People with shingles should avoid cold and get a lot of rest. It's best to keep them isolated, especially if there are children around who have not yet had chickenpox.

Nutrition

Drink only vegetable broth and spring water for two days. Then adopt a hypotoxic diet (see Appendix B) and eliminate eggs, meat, and cheese. Wheat, rice, and barley are recommended foods. Drink a lot of carrot juice, cut down on your salt intake, and opt for foods rich in Vitamin B, especially Vitamin B1. Brewer's yeast and wheat germ are both excellent sources of B vitamins.

Plant Power

Plants can provide wonderful support and relief for people who are fighting off a case of shingles. The three below are highly recommended.

Wallpepper alleviates pain caused by shingles. Obtain fresh sap by putting a few leaves through a blender or extractor, or simply cut the leaves along the horizontal axis; apply the sap to affected areas several times a day.

Soapwort lessens shingles symptoms. To prepare concentrated infusions, use 1 1/2 oz to 2 oz of dried roots per quart of water; let stand for 15 minutes, and apply as compresses.

Marigold (calendula) is very effective for curing a large variety of skin problems. To prepare a marigold tincture, soak a handful of flowers in three times their volume of 40-proof alcohol for 10 days, in direct sunlight or near some other heat source. You can also use compresses dipped in a marigold infusion: Use 1 oz of flowers per quart of water and apply to affected areas.

✍ Sinusitis

Sinusitis simply means an inflammation of the sinus cavities, generally triggered by a nasal or dental infection. The condition often follows a bout of the flu, scarlet fever, or a head cold and is sometimes a symptom of liver problems.

Symptoms of acute sinusitis include a runny nose (usually only one nostril at a time) and pain under the eye on the same side as the affected nostril. Acute sinusitis can become chronic, resulting in persistent nasal secretions, fever, headaches, and a severely limited sense of smell. The condition is also accompanied by frequent colds. If you suspect you are suffering from chronic sinusitis, see a doctor.

General Care

Conventional medical treatments combine antibiotics, inhalations, and anti-inflammatory medications. In some cases nasal puncture and flushing are necessary, both of which are extremely painful. You would be a lot better off using natural remedies to cure or prevent sinusitis. Inhalations help decongest nasal passages, and compresses and baths help alleviate pain.

Chewing pieces of beeswax honeycomb (spit out the wax) decongests nasal passages and alleviates sinus pain. Chew small pieces of honeycomb for a couple of hours, two or three times a day.

Plant Power

If you experience any of the symptoms of sinusitis, try one of the herbal remedies listed below. You may be surprised and pleased with the results.

Chamomile inhalations decongest nasal passages. Add 1 oz of plant to a quart of boiling water, cover your head with a towel or large piece of material, lean over the steaming pot, and inhale the vapor.

Eucalyptus is an antiseptic and expectorant and makes an excellent remedy for respiratory disorders. Use it for inhalations and to fumigate sickrooms. For inhalations, use 3 oz of the plant per quart of boiling water; cover your head with a towel or large piece of material, lean over the steaming pot, and inhale the vapor. You can also combine eucalyptus with thyme (an expectorant that helps reduce fever), pine cones (an antiseptic), and juniper berries (a disinfectant): Mix 1 oz of eucalyptus with 2 oz each of thyme and pine cones; add 2 oz to 3 oz of the mixture to a quart of boiling water and inhale the steaming vapor. To fumigate a sickroom, simply boil some eucalyptus leaves in an uncovered pot in the room.

Fenugreek is an emollient (it soothes inflamed tissues). Use it to prepare poultices: Grind some seeds into powder and mix with a little hot water; apply to inflamed nasal passages when still fairly hot and leave in place for at least 10 minutes.

Lily of the valley decongests nasal passages and alleviates headache pain caused by sinusitis. Grind some dried leaves into powder, using a mortar and pestle, and inhale the powder as snuff. Use three or four pinches a day.

Onion helps decongest blocked nasal passages: Cut an onion into quarters and apply them to the nape of the neck, using a strip of gauze to hold them in place; leave in place overnight.

⇜ Skin Problems

Like your hair and nails, the condition of your skin is a good indication of your overall health. Skin that is marred by lesions or eruptions is often a sign of a more serious health problem. Chronic constipation, for example, can visibly affect your complexion. So to eliminate skin problems related to some other disorder, of course, the underlying cause must be treated first.

WINTER PRECAUTIONS

Winter is hard on your skin, so special care must be taken to protect it. First, reduce the amount of soap you use to wash your face and spread a thin layer of sweet almond or corn oil on your skin after each washing. Don't use too much cologne, which dissolves protective skin oil. St. John's wort oil helps protect the skin against the ravages of winter.

General Care

It's important to understand that taking care of your skin is not simply a matter of applying creams and lotions. You also have to develop lifestyle habits that will promote healthy skin. Here are some ways to do just that.

Take a break from make-up. Over the past few years, manufacturers have become more aware of the importance of using natural substances in makeup, as they're gentler to the skin than are artificially produced, chemical products. Nevertheless, the long-term use of any type of cream, powder, or lotion, organic or not, can obstruct pores, resulting in complexion problems. It's impor-

> ## BEST BETS FOR CLEAN SKIN
>
> The most important aspects of skin care is a thorough daily cleaning that eliminates accumulations of dirt, excess oil, and the fine layer of dead surface skin. Castile or glycerin soap is best for this purpose, and rinsing with water mixed with a little vinegar (cider vinegar has less of an unpleasant odor than ordinary vinegar) helps reestablish the skin's natural pH balance. An occasional cleaning with rose water and the application of natural masks are also helpful for maintaining clear, healthy skin.

tant to give your skin a chance to breathe by not applying cosmetic products for a few days out of every month. Skin that's always covered tends to age prematurely, which is exactly the opposite of what you hope to achieve.

Use sense with scents. Applying too much cologne, perfume, or soap can destroy beneficial bacteria that help keep your skin healthy. That can result in local irritation, especially if you have sensitive skin.

Be careful how you moisturize. If you have dry skin, don't use petroleum jelly or other glycerin-based products. Although they appear to moisturize surface skin, they dry out underlying layers because oil glands in the skin become lazy and inefficient when you do all their work for them.

Take the lipstick test. Some lipsticks dry out your lips and can cause eczema. To test a lipstick, apply a small amount to the skin on your arm and don't wash it away for 24 hours. If you see any redness on your skin, you can conclude that the lipstick in question is not good for your skin type.

Spare the eye shadow. Daily use of eye shadow can cause dermatitis to develop on the eyelids, and ulcers on the cornea. It's better to use it only for special occasions.

Be careful of creams. Even depilatory creams and medical soaps can have an adverse effect on your skin—consult a specialist before using them. Avoid using cortisone-based creams unless specifically prescribed by a doctor. Studies have shown that cortisone creams can cause serious re-infection when used to treat infectious or viral skin problems like shingles or herpes. They also retard healing, bleach the skin around affected areas, promote the appearance of warts, and stimulate the growth of body hair on treated areas of skin.

Nutrition

What you eat plays a huge role in keeping your skin healthy. You can help your complexion by drinking a lot of water between meals. Fruit juice (notably grapefruit) and skim milk (a glass before going to bed at night) are also recommended. Foods like carrots, pork, liver, eggs, fresh water fish, celery, cauliflower, endive, spinach, dandelion, parsley, chicory, citrus fruit, pineapple, bananas, and apples all contain vitamins and other nutrients that benefit your skin.

Don't drink a lot while eating, and avoid spicy foods, alcohol, coffee, greasy foods, or fat sauces. Also remember that ingesting excessive amounts of salt can cause skin problems.

Vitamin Power

Where your skin is concerned, the vitamins and minerals you put into your body are far more powerful than plant remedies. Here are the nutrients that will give you the healthiest, most vibrant skin you can have.

Vitamin A is important for the skin, hair, eyes, teeth, and nails. It helps keep your skin young looking, and prevents pimples and other types of skin eruptions. A deficiency results in dilated pores and scaly skin that cracks easily. Good sources of Vitamin A include carrots, tomatoes, leafy green vegetables, watercress, parsley, and dandelion.

Vitamin B has a beneficial effect on your general health and helps keep your skin looking young by preventing the formation of wrinkles, especially on the face. Good sources include wheat germ, brewer's yeast, brown rice, and yogurt.

Vitamin C promotes healing and prevents infection. A Vitamin C-rich diet helps keep your skin supple and firm. A deficiency results in skin dis-

SKIN CANCER

There are different forms of skin cancer, the two main types being carcinoma and malignant melanoma.

Carcinoma-type cancer generally appears on areas of skin that are frequently exposed to light. Basal cell carcinoma almost always appears on the face, and especially around the nose. The initial symptom is a small ulcer that is slightly darker than the color of the skin. The ulcer develops into a plaque with small bumps around the edge and becomes covered with scales that detach easily.

Spino-cellular carcinoma generally affects persons over the age of 40 and appears on skin that has been damaged by disease, burns, etc. A small growth that tends to bleed easily appears first. It then spreads, forming more growths. Prolonged and systematic exposure of the skin to direct sunlight is a contributing cause of this type of cancer.

Malignant melanoma cancers usually begin growing around beauty spots that are frequently rubbed or irritated in some other fashion. They are more dangerous than carcinoma-type skin cancers. Don't touch beauty spots or other marks on your skin, in order to prevent them from degenerating into melanoma-type cancer.

If you detect any of the symptoms listed below, see a doctor as soon as possible—rapid surgical intervention is the only way to cure skin cancer at present. Although plants can help prevent skin cancer and alleviate symptoms in some cases, they cannot cure the disease. Like all treatments, plants have their limits.

Symptoms to Look For:
- Moles that start to bleed
- Moles that increase in size
- Moles that turn black or a combination of colors (brown, black, red, etc.)
- The appearance of a reddish ring around a mole
- Moles with an uneven shape or notched or jagged edges

coloration, loss of skin tone, and the formation of wrinkles. Good sources of Vitamin C include cabbage, potatoes, cauliflower, strawberries, lemons and other citrus fruits, green peppers, and kiwi fruit.

Vitamin D is produced by the skin when exposed to sunlight and is destroyed by alkaline soaps. Good dietary sources of Vitamin D include butter and cheese, herring, mackerel, algae, almonds, pineapple, and oats.

Vitamin E accelerates healing, tones the skin by stimulating circulation, and prevents varicose veins. Good sources include wheat germ and wheat germ oil, sunflower seed oil, soya oil, sprouted wheat, and watercress.

Minerals are extremely important to skin health, especially calcium, phosphorous, iron, iodine, silicon, sulfur, and magnesium. Good sources of these minerals include turnips, onions, asparagus, radishes, brussels sprouts, lettuce, carrots, leeks, and potatoes.

❧ Sore Throat

Anything from mouth breathing to infection can cause that raw, stinging, burning sensation in our throats that can make eating, talking, and even plain old swallowing difficult. The good news is that you don't have to put up with the discomfort.

Plant Power

Of course, the shelves at the local pharmacy are loaded with lozenges and pain killers—usually made with lots of sugar and artificial chemicals. But if you'd rather treat the pain with natural remedies that will encourage healing rather than simply deadening the nerves in your throat, try some of the plants listed below.

Agrimony is recommended for treating mouth sores, hoarseness, and angina. Boil 3 oz of leaves in a quart of water for 15 minutes, filter, and cool. Use the liquid as a gargle. This remedy can also help you clear your voice before speaking in public.

Cayenne helps alleviate pain. Add a pinch of powder to a cup of boiling water, cool, and use the liquid as a gargle.

Marjoram should be used as an external treatment, to alleviate pain caused by a sore throat during the night. Prepare a concentrated marjoram infusion: 2 oz of flowers and leaves per quart of water; let stand for 10 minutes. Soak a strip of cotton in the liquid and wrap around the throat, as tightly as possible without causing discomfort. Cover with a strip of flannel.

Walnut contains a natural antibiotic and can be used as a gargle and mouthwash. To prepare concentrated infusions, add 1 oz of leaves to a quart of boiling water.

Apple cider vinegar can be used as an external treatment: Soak a strip of cotton in the cider vinegar and wrap it around the neck; cover with a strip of wool or flannel.

Thyme has antiseptic properties that make it an effective remedy for sore throats, head colds, and bronchitis. Use 1 oz per quart of water to prepare infusions, and sweeten with honey to soothe a sore throat.

Rose is an astringent and antiseptic. Its mildly anaesthetizing effect helps alleviate pain caused by throat inflammation. Prepare concentrated infusions: 1 1/2 oz to 2 oz of petals per quart of water, to be used as a gargle.

Blackberry leaves contain a lot of tannin and organic acid, making it an effective treatment for mouth, gum, and throat inflammation. Boil 2 oz to 3 oz of leaves in a quart of water for 10 minutes. Cool and use as a gargle.

≫ Sprains

Sprains are the most common of all acute sports injuries in the United States. They occur when a foot gets turned the wrong way or somebody steps on it accidentally and ligaments in the ankle tear. That can result in anything from local tenderness to swelling, bruising, and an inability to stand on the injured ankle.

Plant Power

Fortunately, most sprain injuries are of the local type and don't require major medical intervention. If you find yourself with this kind of injury—and it can happen during any activity from bowling to taking a walk—try some of the plant remedies listed below to help you heal.

Arnica is recommended for all types of injuries that have not produced open wounds. Dilute 2/3 oz of arnica tincture in 1 1/2 oz of glycerin. To prepare your own tincture, place 1 1/2 oz of flowers in one cup of 60-proof alcohol; soak for 10 days, agitating the liquid from time to time; press through a coffee filter and store in a sealed container; dilute just before applying.

FIRST AID FOR MINOR SPRAINS

The word to remember for many sports or activity related injuries is RICE. It stands for rest, ice, compression, and elevation.

Rest: Don't use the injured body part! If it's an ankle, stop walking on it. It's already been stressed enough.

Ice: Apply ice to the area for several hours, but be sure and wrap it in cloth so that you won't get freeze damage to your skin. You can try a 20-minutes-on, 20-minutes-off routine if the cold feels too extreme.

Compression: Put an elastic bandage on the injured part. Along with the ice, that will help to keep swelling down.

Elevation: Elevate the sprain either on pillows or in a sling.

After the first 24 hours, you can stop using ice and apply heat (hot water bottle or heating pad) instead. Stay off the injured joint until it's completely healed. If there's discoloration or the joint looks oddly shaped, see a doctor.

Ginger infusions, added to your bath water, stimulate circulation and alleviate pain. Use 1/3 oz of plant per quart of water to prepare infusions, and add enough to your bath to turn the water slightly yellow.

Onion can be applied directly to the affected joint to help accelerate healing.

Marigold works wonderfully as a lotion to accelerate healing. Boil 2/3 oz of petals in one cup of milk; remove from heat, and let stand for three hours; filter and apply directly to affected joints.

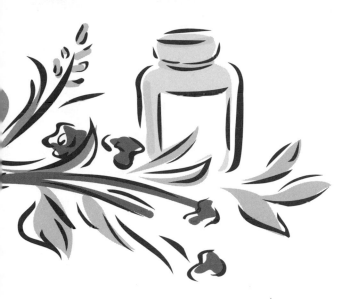

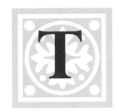

✐ Teething Pain
(Infant)

This period of childhood is one most parents could do without. Not only is teething painful, but it can also cause fever, bronchitis, and earaches (which just goes to show how closely various parts of the body are interrelated). It's no surprise that teething infants are often agitated, even when being held, and become exhausted from lack of sleep.

Plant Power

Teething is unpleasant, but both parents and children can get through it more easily with some help from the plants listed on page 220.

BABY TEETHING TIMETABLE

Teething, like everything else in a baby's schedule, will happen at nature's convenience, not yours. But this will give you a general idea of when you can expect teeth to show up.

Upper:
- Front incisors—8–13 months
- Side incisors—8–13 months
- Canines (cuspids)—16–23 months
- First molars—13–19 months
- Second molars—25–33 months

Lower:
- Front incisors—6–10 months
- Side incisors—10–16 months
- Canines (cuspids)—16–23 months
- First molars—13–19 months
- Second molars—23–31 months

Plantain tincture helps soothe pain caused by teething. Rub directly on the child's gums.

Marshmallow root can be given to infants to suck on. It rapidly alleviates gum inflammation and helps new teeth break through. Make certain that you hold the root while your baby is sucking to avoid any problems with choking.

❧ Testicle Swelling and Pain

Orchitis is the medical term for inflammation of the testicles. Usually the testicles swell, and the scrotum takes on a reddish color. High fever and intense pain are hallmarks. A doctor will prescribe antibiotics to treat the problem, but homeopathic remedies can also be helpful.

General Care

During the acute stage patients should stay in bed, with testicles raised above the thighs (use a piece of cardboard to hold them up) to alleviate pain. If pain is very intense, apply an ice pack to the testicles, which should be wrapped in a piece of flannel.

TESTICULAR SELF-EXAM

Testicular cancer is the most common type of cancer in males between the ages of 15 and 35, but with early detection, 9 out of 10 people can be cured of it.

In the same way women do self-exams of their breasts, you should do a testicular self-exam once a month, preferably after a warm bath or shower. Here's how to do it.

Stand naked in front of a mirror. Look for any swelling or unusual shapes in the scrotum. If one testicle is larger than the other, don't worry. That's normal.

Place the index and middle fingers of both hands on the top of one testicle. Now roll it gently between your thumbs and fingers. If you find a pea-sized, painless lump on the front or side, it's time to see a doctor. You should be aware that there is a tube connected to the top and back of the testicle called the epididymis. It is not a lump and should not worry you.

Plant Power

As painful—and perhaps frightening—as this condition may be, don't panic. There is plenty of help available among the herbal remedies listed here.

White dead nettle decongests inflamed tissues. Throughout the course of the day, drink infusions, prepared with 2/3 oz of flowers per quart of water.

Malva is another plant that decongests inflamed tissues. Drink infusions throughout the day: 2/3 oz of flowers per quart of water.

St. John's wort oil can help soothe painful testicles: Soak 1 lb of freshly picked flowers in half a quart of olive oil and half a quart of white wine; boil the wine off in a double boiler, filter, and cool.

❧ Tobacco Addiction

Everybody knows that smoking causes cancer and heart attacks. And everybody knows they should quit. Unfortunately, that's easier said than done.

The problem with addictions is that you really don't want to give them up. That's what makes them addictions. So if you want to throw away the cigarettes for good, the first thing you've got to do is develop a sincere desire to quit. Once you've done that, there's no way you can fail.

Whether to stop all at once or gradually wean yourself off cigarettes will be your next decision. If you've been a heavy smoker for a number of years, reducing the number of cigarettes you smoke by half is already a step in the right direction. But whatever method you choose, you'll probably need help. Here are some guidelines you may find useful.

Keep a count. Instead of lighting up whenever you feel the urge, keep a careful count of the number of cigarettes you smoke each day. Counting acts as a psychological barrier and will automatically reduce your tobacco consumption.

Wait awhile. Try to postpone lighting your first cigarette a little longer each day, and never lose sight of your goal, which is to quit, or at least drastically reduce the number of cigarettes you smoke. When you do have your first cigarette, make a note of the time and circumstances; for example, 10

WHY IS IT SO HARD TO QUIT SMOKING?

To nonsmokers, just the smell of a cigarette can be nauseating. So why do smokers have such a hard time giving up the habit? According to some recent research, the answer may lie deep within the brain. Studies have shown that significant changes occur in the brain's pleasure circuits when you try to quit smoking. These changes are very similar to those seen during withdrawal from cocaine, heroin, amphetamines, and alcohol. When you abruptly withdraw from one of these substances, your brain seems to lose its ability to experience pleasure. These changes can last for days and may even cause depression and anxiety. The good news is that with persistence and patience, your brain soon returns to normal and your smoking can become a thing of the past.

A.M., after breakfast, or 12 P.M., after lunch (it's a good idea to buy a little note pad specifically for this purpose). Make it a kind of personal challenge to extend the time before lighting your first cigarette each day. Also note down how you feel before and after you light up (light-headed, easier breathing, dizzy, etc.).

Be fickle. Change cigarette brands frequently. Alternate between dark or blonde, menthol, or extra light, etc. This will help diminish the pleasure you get from smoking.

Take time off. Try to go without smoking at least one day a week. Then stop for a whole week, then two weeks, then a whole month, etc. Do this gradually, say over a period of two years.

Distract yourself. When you feel the urge to smoke, do something else instead: Eat a carrot or a celery stalk, drink a glass of water, suck a candy, or give your teeth a good brushing.

Plant Power

What better way to fight the urge for a harmful herb—tobacco—than to use healthy ones? Here are some that can be your allies in your fight to quit smoking.

Watercress is an antidote for nicotine. People who smoke would do well to consume large amounts of this plant. Gargling with watercress juice reinforces the gums and combats bad breath. Use a juice extractor or a mortar and pestle to obtain fresh sap and mix with a little water.

Hedge mustard alleviates the need to smoke. Infuse 1 oz in a quart of boiled water for 10 minutes and drink a cup in the morning before breakfast and another before going to bed at night.

Sweet flag induces mild nausea in smokers, making them less likely to want to light up. Simply chew on some fresh root during the course of the day.

Coltsfoot makes a good substitute for tobacco and at the same time helps combat coughing. Simply roll the dried leaves into cigarettes.

☜ Tonsillitis

Tonsillitis should not be confused with other types of sore throat. The condition, characterized by inflammation of the tonsils (tiny glands located in the throat), can be either acute or chronic and generally requires medical attention.

If the following symptoms appear, immediate intervention is necessary: intense pain, high fever, extremely sore throat, swollen tonsil glands, the appearance of a membrane or white spots on the tonsil glands (in which case the condition may not be tonsillitis but angina, caused by diphtheria).

Any plant remedies you use should be fast-acting and applied as early as possible. Once the problem has become acute, medical intervention is generally a must. Persons suffering from tonsillitis should stay in bed as long as they continue to run a fever.

Nutrition

Milk and other dairy products, fruit juices, vegetable broth, stewed vegetables, and crackers are all recommended. Avoid eating bread and other starchy foods and use as little salt as possible.

Older children and adults can add sources of magnesium to their diet. These include whole grains, potatoes, fish, oysters, and hard white cheese.

Plant Power

Although you may need to be in the care of a doctor, there are some things you can do at home to help you cope with this condition. Here are some remedies to try.

Burdock infusions (1 oz in a quart of boiling water, infused for 5 or 10 minutes, then cooled) make an excellent gargle.

Mallow acts as a decongestant and helps fight inflammation. Prepare the remedy cold: Soak a heaping teaspoon in a cup of water overnight. The next morning, heat slightly and drink three or four cups a day, a mouthful at a time.

Sage also makes an effective gargle: Soak a heaping teaspoon of leaves (picked before the plant has had a chance to flower if possible) in a cup of cold water for about half an hour. You can also use a sage infusion (a heaping teaspoon of leaves per cup of water) to gargle after it has cooled, or soak some gauze in the liquid and apply directly to the inflamed tonsils. *Note: Do not use this remedy on very young children.*

Tumors (Benign)

Like cancer tumors, benign tumors are masses of cells that form into growths, but they don't spread or grow out of control. Still, because they take up so much space, they can cause various problems and usually need to be removed through surgery. Natural remedies can shrink tumors and have provided encouraging results in many cases, but that doesn't mean you should avoid consulting a doctor. If you think you're developing a tumor, get it diagnosed as soon as possible. If the tumor is cancerous, diagnosis and treatment are critical.

Plant Power

Before trying any of the plants below, makes sure you get your doctor's okay. Some herbal remedies can reduce the effectiveness of certain drug therapies. But used in conjunction with your doctor's treatment, home remedies may provide a valuable secondary support for the therapy he or she recommends.

St. John's wort oil can be combined with the humble potato to combat tumors. The treatment takes some time to work, so be patient. Day one: Boil some potatoes in their peel, then mash and mix with a little milk; apply hot or cold to affected areas. Day two: Apply hot cabbage leaf compresses (remove the sides and large veins). Day three: Apply a mixture of St. John's wort oil and horsetail infusion. To prepare your own St. John's wort oil, fill a container with fresh leaves (don't pack too tightly), cover with extra virgin olive oil, seal the container, and let stand in direct sunlight or near some other heat source; when the oil turns red, filter through a piece of cloth.

Plantain was a sacred plant of the ancient druids. It is supposed to help reduce tumors and other types of skin swelling; apply some plantain paste to affected areas: Simply wash some fresh leaves and crush them with a rolling pin while still wet.

Horsetail helps inhibit the growth of tumors, especially when combined with a depurative remedy. Heat horsetail leaves in a double boiler, then wrap them in some linen and apply to the affected area; leave in place for two hours, three times a day (every day), morning, noon, and night. Also drink a cup of horsetail decoction in the morning a half hour before breakfast, and another before your evening meal: Boil 1 1/2 oz to 2 oz of plant in a quart of water for half an hour.

Marigold (calendula) also combats tumors. Use marigold along with a depurative remedy and horsetail. Combine the following herbs and drink 1 1/2 quarts to 2 quarts a day: 10 oz of marigold flowers, 3 oz of yarrow, and 3 oz of nettle. Use the mixture to prepare six cups of infusion, adding a few drops of gooseberry juice to each; wait at least one hour between cups.

Thyme baths revitalize fatigued organisms: Boil 1 lb of plant in two quarts of water for 15 minutes and add the decoction to your bath water. Thyme also helps combat edema, which often occurs during the treatment of tumors. Use 1 oz of plant per quart of water to prepare infusions and drink four or five cups a day.

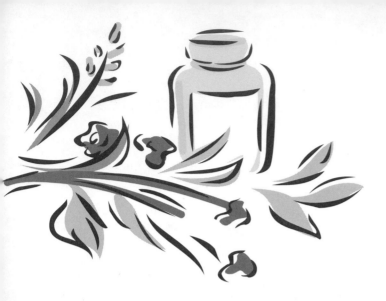

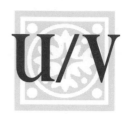

🌿 Ulcers (Skin and Mucosa)

Say the word "ulcer" and most people immediately think of the stomach, but the fact is that many ulcers affect the skin or mucous membranes and have nothing to do with the stomach. Chronic ulcers, in the form of oozing eruptions, usually appear on the legs.

An ulcer is simply any lesion on the skin or a mucous membrane that forms pus and is surrounded by dead tissue.

Plant Power

Plants are very helpful for treating ulcers, for two reasons: They keep the lesions clean, and they accelerate the healing process. Here are some to try.

Burdock makes a very effective external application: Crush some fresh leaves in a mortar and pestle and apply directly to affected areas. You can also soak the crushed leaves in olive oil and put them in direct sunlight or near some other heat source for 24 hours. Apply daily (this remedy can be preserved for only a few days).

Cow parsnip alleviates swelling around ulcers: Apply freshly ground leaves and roots to affected areas.

Lavender is an antiseptic that accelerates healing. Use decoctions or tinctures to prepare compresses. Decoctions require 1 oz of lavender flowers per quart of water. To prepare your own lavender tincture, soak 1 1/2 oz of flowers in a cup of 30-proof alcohol for two weeks.

Malva is an emollient (soothes inflammation) that also reduces swelling. Prepare compresses with a concentrated decoction of leaves or roots: 1 oz to 1 1/2 oz per quart of water.

Walnut accelerates healing and combats infection. Use decoctions to prepare compresses: Use between 1 1/2 oz and 2 oz of leaves per quart of water.

Plantain alleviates inflammation and accelerates healing. Wash the leaves in some boiling water for a few seconds before grinding them with a mortar and pestle; apply directly to affected areas. You can also prepare compresses using a plantain decoction: Boil 1 oz to 2 oz of the plant in a quart of water for three minutes, then remove from heat and let stand for three minutes.

Silverweed compresses are astringent (they help tissues contract). Prepare decoctions using 1 oz to 2 oz per quart of water.

Horsetail decoctions make an effective dressing for ulcerated skin: Boil 1 oz to 2 oz of dried plant in a quart of water for half an hour.

Thyme cleans and disinfects ulcers, and soothes pain. Use concentrated decoctions to bathe affected areas and prepare compresses: Boil 3 oz of the plant in a quart of water until half the water has evaporated.

Coltsfoot is recommended for tubercular ulcers and lesions that become ulcerated. To treat tubercular ulcers, drink five or six cups of decoction a day: 1 oz per quart of water. For ulcerated lesions, crush some fresh leaves and apply as a poultice to reduce inflammation and accelerate healing.

≈ Ulcers (Stomach and Duodenal)

Ulcers that appear on the wall of the stomach (peptic) or small bowel gradually eat away the mucous membranes lining these organs. Potential causes include work-related stress, abuse of certain medications (aspirin, corticoids), an improper diet, or perhaps most commonly, a bacteria called *helicobacter pylori*.

The pain associated with peptic ulcers becomes most intense a few hours after meals. Eating tends to alleviate it, except if the food is very spicy. As the ulcer develops, attacks occur more frequently. Or they may stop after a

SYMPTOMS OF AN ULCER

How do you know if you have an ulcer? Here are some of the signs your body may give you.

- Stomach very hard and permanently contracted
- Severe pain in the abdominal region, as if you've just taken a punch to the stomach
- Black stool and red or black vomit (an indication of internal bleeding)

Don't ignore these symptoms if they occur—see a doctor as soon as possible.

few weeks, only to recur some months later.

Pain from duodenal (small bowel) ulcers, which usually begins five or six hours after eating, can be very severe and usually requires medical attention.

If you think you have an ulcer, see a doctor. The condition can be very serious—complications from a peptic ulcer can result in a perforated stomach, internal bleeding, or cancer. Duodenal ulcer complications include internal bleeding and the shrinking of part of the intestine.

THE ULCER-FIGHTING LIFESTYLE

The discovery of the *H. pylori* bacteria as the major cause of stomach ulcers in humans has turned antibiotics into one of our most powerful tools for restoring digestive health, but it's not the only one. We still need to mind our lifestyle and avoid anything that might aggravate an existing ulcer or weaken our immune defense against new ones. Here are some tips to remember.

- Take your time when you sit down for a meal, and make sure to chew your food well.
- Avoid heated discussions at mealtime, and don't read or watch TV while eating.
- Avoid spicy foods, soft drinks, very hot soup, and hot liquids in general.
- Don't drink a lot of liquids while you eat. The liquids you do drink should be at room temperature.
- Reduce your salt intake.
- Avoid aspirin and cortisone-based medications.
- Start your meals with a glass of freshly pressed potato and cabbage juice. You can also add some of the juice to your soup if you enjoy the taste.
- After each meal, drink a glass of water with a teaspoon of powdered charcoal dissolved in it.
- Replace bicarbonate of soda with dried raw oat flakes.

Nutrition

Try to adopt a healthy, well-balanced diet. Avoid coffee and alcohol as much as possible. Best bets for food include bananas, carrots, fresh pineapple, and lavender or rosemary honey.

Plant Power

Mother Nature has devoted a large section of her garden to plants that can help you cope with stomach ulcers. Try some of the ones listed here.

Almonds help inhibit the production of pepsin, a major protein component of gastric juices that are over-secreted by stomachs affected by an ulcer. They also improve intestinal functions and create a protective layer around the stomach lining. Eat about 2 oz of peeled almonds, twice a day. You can also mix chopped almonds in a cup of milk and half a cup of fresh cream, and add a bitter almond if the ulcer persists.

Cabbage helps heal ulcers. Eat a lot of raw cabbage and take one or two teaspoons of cabbage juice a day, obtained by putting some leaves through an extractor or blender.

Geranium helps rebuild a damaged stomach lining. Drink a cup of decoction before your midday and evening meals: Soak 1 1/2 oz of the plant in a quart of cold water for 10 minutes, then slowly bring to a boil for two minutes; remove from heat and let stand for another 10 minutes.

Hops soothe stomach inflammation, alleviate spasms, and have a calming, sedative effect when taken in large doses. The plant is recommended for ulcers related to nervousness. Use 1/2 oz of cones per quart of water to prepare infusions, and drink three or four cups a day.

RECIPES FOR A HAPPY STOMACH

If you have a peptic ulcer, here are two great herbal recipes that can ease your pain and jump start your recovery.

Herbal mixture #1: 1 oz of marigold, 1 1/2 oz of knotgrass; mix the ingredients, then boil a teaspoon in a cup of water for a few minutes; remove from heat and infuse for 10 minutes; filter, and sip three or four cups a day.

Herbal mixture #2: 25 grams of marshmallow, 25 grams of licorice, 1 1/2 oz of comfrey, and 1 oz of hops; boil six tablespoons of the mixture in a quart of water, then remove from heat and infuse for 20 minutes; drink five or six cups a day, between meals.

Malva has a soothing effect on the stomach and calms inflammation of mucous membranes. The plant is often mixed with barley: Cook the barley, cool, and add some malva leaves to prepare a delicious and beneficial meal.

Potatoes are amazingly beneficial for the stomach, acting as an antacid and emollient and accelerating healing. It is recommended for the treatment of ulcers and excess acidity. Drink four glasses of raw potato juice a day (add a little lemon to taste).

Licorice can cure stomach ulcers and, in some cases, duodenal ulcers as well. The plant covers the stomach wall with a viscous protective layer that reduces acidic secretions and accelerates healing of lesions. It also has a relaxing, anti-inflammatory and antispasmodic effect. Use 1 oz of plant per quart of water to prepare infusions and drink three to five cups a day.

Note that persons with high blood pressure, heart problems, or paralysis problems should not use licorice for a prolonged period of time.

Sweet flag is recommended for the treatment of duodenal ulcers. Soak a teaspoon of root in two cups of cold water overnight; reheat in a double boiler before drinking and take one teaspoon before meals (not more than six teaspoons a day).

❧ Uremia

Urea is a by-product of your body's breaking down proteins. Too much urea in the blood (more than two grams per quart) causes a condition known as uremia. The problem is usually linked to poor kidney function.

Plant Power

Medicinal plants such as the ones listed here can help control and cure this condition.

Couchgrass (also called doggrass) is a depurative and diuretic that alleviates inflammation of the urinary tract. Boil 1 oz of chopped rhizomes in 1-1/2 quarts of water for one minute; discard the water and boil again in a quart of water for 15 minutes; add a zest of lemon and a bit of licorice to taste; then cool. Filter, and drink a quart a day.

THE TELLTALE SIGNS OF UREMIA

The symptoms listed here could mean many things, but if they mean uremia, you'll need rapid treatment. If you experience any of these signs, consult a doctor as soon as possible.

- Frequent headaches
- Persistent cramps and pain in various parts of the body
- Prickling sensations in the limbs and extremities
- Loss of appetite, nausea, vomiting
- Memory loss and extreme fatigue

Symptoms of acute uremia include a marked pallor, general swelling, and loss of appetite. An artificial kidney or a kidney transplant is sometimes the only way to cure the condition.

Common broom is a powerful diuretic that helps purify the blood and eliminate waste. Boil 1 oz to 2 oz of stems in a quart of water for a few minutes, then remove from heat and infuse for 10 minutes. Drink five or six cups a day.

Common hawkweed (sometimes called mouse ear) helps eliminate urea and regulates the level of urea in the blood. It also fights infections and stimulates liver functions. Use 1 oz to 2 oz of dried leaves per quart of water to prepare infusions, and drink two or three cups a day.

Linden is recommended for cases of uremia. Use 1 oz of flowers per quart of water to

THE UREMIA-BUSTING DIET

The way you eat can have a profound effect on this condition. In general, reduce your intake of bread, meat, and fish to 2 oz of one or the other a day. Also cut down on your salt intake.

Then try the following regimen, to be followed one week per month: one day of potatoes and fat; one day of fruit and vegetables; one day of rice, fruit, and sugar. Alternate until the week is over. For the rest of the month, adopt a hypotoxic diet composed of legumes, cauliflower, fruit, vegetables (except spinach and sorrel); 3 oz of meat or white fish a day, or an egg and a cup of milk; drink as much spring water and herbal infusion as you like; cut down on coffee, tea, and red wine and eliminate white wine and hard liquor completely.

prepare infusions and drink three or four cups a day for a prolonged period of time.

〰 Urethritis

If you've ever had urethritis, you know it. It's an inflammation of the urethra, the tube through which urine is evacuated from the bladder, that causes an intense, burning pain while urinating. The infection can come from gonococcal bacteria, in which case the condition is known as gonorrheal or venereal urethritis.

In some cases, pain spreads to the kidneys and is accompanied by fever. Urine flow becomes weak and may contain discharge.

This disorder needs fast treatment, especially in women, because complications can be serious. There is also a risk of sterility for both sexes. Consult a doctor who will conduct tests to confirm the diagnosis.

General Care

Conventional treatments are based on antibiotics and diuretics. Otherwise, here is what to do.

Abstain from sex. It is obviously best to abstain from sexual relations until the condition has been cured, especially during the acute phase. Be frank and tell your partner(s) about the problem.

Rest. Avoid getting overly fatigued, and don't embark on any long trips by car, bus, or train.

Soothe with warmth. Take frequent baths in lukewarm water. It will help ease the discomfort.

Keep your hands down. Avoid touching your face with your hands, and keep your hands as clean as possible, especially after urinating.

Watch your diet. Eat a lot of fruit and drink fruit juices. Avoid alcohol, which irritates the urinary tract.

Plant Power

Diuretic and antiseptic plant remedies can be extremely effective for treating this problem. They can prevent the spread of bacteria and regenerate mucous membranes damaged by the disease, reducing the risk of a recurrence. Here are the best ones to use.

Boldo is an antiseptic that is recommended for cases of chronic urethritis and urinary and genital disorders in general. Use 1/3 oz of leaves per quart of water to prepare infusions (add a little fresh mint to increase the plant's effectiveness) and drink a cup before meals.

Borage is a powerful diuretic. Use 1 oz of flowers per quart of boiled water to prepare infusions, and drink three or four cups a day.

Shepherd's purse is an antiseptic for the urinary tract. To prevent recurrences, drink infusions after the infection has cleared up.

Bearberry is an effective diuretic and antiseptic for the urinary tract (don't worry if urine takes on a brownish color). Use 1 oz of dried leaves per quart of water to prepare infusions, and drink three or four cups a day.

Eucalyptus is an antiseptic that is very effective for combating urinary infections. Prepare infusions using 1 oz of leaves per quart of water and drink four or five cups a day. You can also combine 1 oz of eucalyptus with 2/3 oz of bearberry and 2/3 oz of broom heather; add a tablespoon of the mixture to a cup of cold water; bring to a boil, remove from heat, and infuse for 10 minutes; drink three cups a day, morning, noon, and night, between meals.

Juniper berries are diuretic and antiseptic and are recommended for all types of urinary disorders. Use 1 oz of dried crushed berries per quart of water to prepare infusions and drink two or three cups a day, between meals. You can also drink infusions after the condition has cleared up to prevent recurrences. *Important Note: Pregnant women and persons suffering from kidney problems should not use this remedy.*

Parsley is a depurative and diuretic that is very effective for treating urethritis and other urinary tract infections. Drink a tablespoon of fresh parsley juice every morning before breakfast (use an extractor or crush some parsley leaves in a mortar and pestle and then press through a fine cloth to obtain your juice).

Pine is a diuretic and antiseptic that is recommended for treating bladder and urinary infections. Infuse 1 oz of buds in a quart of water, sweeten with honey, and drink three or four cups a day.

Goldenrod has the same effect as shepherd's purse and other antiseptics. It's also an astringent (contracts tissues), diuretic, and anti-inflammatory. Pour a quart of boiling water over 1/2 oz of flower tops, infuse for a few minutes, and drink three cups a day.

SPRING WATER CURE FOR CYSTITIS

Drinking large amounts of pure spring water can be very helpful for eliminating accumulations of urine where colon bacilli tend to propagate. Try to get your water directly from a natural source instead of buying bottled spring water, which often contains minerals that cannot be assimilated and form deposits in the body. If you have to buy your water, choose a brand with the lowest possible mineral content.

Urinary Colibacillosis

This term refers to infections of the digestive system caused by a bacteria known as colon bacilli, which sometimes spreads to the urinary tract and gallbladder.

If you develop a urinary infection (cystitis), you should consult a doctor. Antibiotics are generally prescribed to cure the problem.

Nutrition

Adopt a hypotoxic diet. If possible, go on a liquid diet for a few days, drinking only spring water, natural fruit juice, and vegetable broth.

When you start ingesting solid food again, make sure your diet includes large amounts of lettuce, raw sauerkraut, grated beets, cucumbers, apples, and blueberries (if you can get them). Avoid coffee, tea, and soft drinks, as well as milk, sugar, fat cheese, and yogurt until you are fully recovered.

Plant Power

As with other problems in the urinary tract, plants can offer powerful healing effects for people with this condition. Try the remedies below.

Broom heather is both a diuretic and an antiseptic for the urinary tract. For that reason it is often prescribed for cases of colon bacilli, usually in conjunction with sweet woodruff, which increases the volume of urine and prevents the spread of the infection. Start with a decoction: Boil 1 oz of broom heather in a quart of water until a third of the water has evaporated; remove from heat and add 1/2 oz of sweet woodruff; drink three cups a day.

Eucalyptus is an effective antiseptic. Boil three or four leaves per cup of water for three minutes, remove from heat and let stand for 10 minutes; drink three cups a day.

Bilberry (also called whortleberry) is useful for treating intestinal infections and cystitis. You can eat the berries themselves or prepare a decoction using the leaves: Boil 1 tablespoon of leaves per cup of water for five minutes.

Goldenrod helps drain the liver and kidneys. This diuretic effect is very helpful for cases of colon bacilli or cystitis. Boil 1 1/2 oz of flower tops in a quart of water for 10 minutes, then remove from heat and let stand for 12 hours; filter and drink over a period of two days.

✎ Urinary Disorders (General)

Almost any change in the color or volume of your urine is a signal of something new going on within your body. Any change that is very unusual, such as blood in the urine, should be brought to a doctor's attention immediately. Changes in color, if persistent, should also be evaluated by a medical professional.

Changes in volume or frequency are also important. For men, urine retention is often caused by the presence of a benign tumor of the prostate (BPH or benign prostatic hyperplasia) and can result in a urinary infection. There is also the chance that it could be caused by a cancerous tumor, so diagnosis is very important.

Plant Power

The curative plants listed below can help control such symptoms as urine retention or insufficient volume of urine.

Bearberry is a diuretic and powerful antiseptic for the urinary tract. If you use this plant, don't worry if your urine takes on a brownish color—it's perfectly normal. Use 1 oz of dried leaves per quart of water to prepare infusions and drink three or four cups a day, between meals.

Eucalyptus is an antiseptic that effectively combats urinary infections. You can also combine this plant with bearberry and broom heather: Mix 2/3 oz of bearberry, 1 oz of broom heather, and 1 oz of eucalyptus; add a tablespoon of

WHAT YOUR URINE CAN TELL YOU

Here are some of the changes you may see in your urine and what those changes may mean:

- Urine can turn green or bluish after being treated with methyline or quinine.
- Bright yellow urine occurs after a prolonged Vitamin C or B12 cure.
- Brownish urine indicates the presence of blood, hemoglobin, or toxins (bearberry infusions can also produce brownish urine). Urine that contains blood can indicate a kidney, bladder, or prostate problem.
- Black urine also indicates the presence of blood. It can also occur after a bout of indigestion or after eating a lot of spinach.
- Whitish urine may contain pus or phosphate. Pus can be a symptom of flu, cystitis, urethritis, a kidney abscess, or septicemia.
- Urine may smell like cat's urine after drinking regular infusions of wild pansy.
- Urine that has a very strong unpleasant odor may indicate a colibacillus infection, cystitis, or a kidney stone.
- Difficulty urinating as well as cloudy urine that contains red or white sediment can be related to gout, a condition called uricemia, or kidney stones.
- A burning sensation while urinating is an indication of urethritis.

the mixture to a cup of boiling water, remove from heat and infuse for 10 minutes; drink three cups a day, morning, noon, and night, between meals.

Fennel is a diuretic that alleviates urine retention and abnormally small urine volume. Infuse 1 oz to 2 oz of roots in a quart of water for one hour and drink three or four cups a day.

Ash is a diuretic that combats problems of urine retention and reduces the amount of uric acid in the blood. Use 1 oz to 1 1/2 oz of leaves per quart of water to prepare infusions and drink three or four cups a day.

Onion in external applications helps combat urine retention. Use onion pulp to prepare poultices that you apply to the lower stomach region. Onions are also diuretic: Eat a raw onion every day.

Parsley is a diuretic and depurative that is recommended for the treatment of all types of urinary disorders. Drink a tablespoon of freshly pressed parsley juice every morning before breakfast. Use an extractor to obtain your juice, or crush some leaves in a mortar and pestle, then add a little water and press through a fine cloth.

Pine is also an effective diuretic and antiseptic that helps cure bladder and urinary tract infections. Infuse 1 oz in a quart of water for half an hour, sweeten with honey to neutralize the bitter taste, and drink three or four cups a day.

Apple helps cure problems of urine retention as well as bladder and urinary tract infections. Dry some apple peel and then crush it into powder; boil a tablespoon of the powder in a cup of water for 15 minutes; add a couple of apple slices and a zest of lemon to taste, and drink three cups a day.

Thyme is a diuretic and antiseptic that makes an effective remedy for urinary tract and intestinal disorders. Use 1/2 oz to 1 oz per quart of water to prepare infusions (do not boil this plant) and drink four or five cups a day.

❧ Vaginal Discharge

We may not exactly like to talk about them, but the fact is that some types of vaginal discharge are quite normal. They're actually uterine secretions that occur during ovulation, or the overly rapid renewal of cells lining the vaginal wall.

Other types of discharge, however, can signal a problem. If you notice a yellowish or greenish color, or an unpleasant odor accompanied by itching or burning sensations, you may have an inflammation of the vagina or cervix.

Vaginal inflammation can result from microscopic organisms, such as fungi or bacteria, and produce a variety of symptoms, including burning sensations, difficulty urinating, and an inability to have sexual relations.

Discharge resulting from inflammation of the cervix is yellowish in color, thick and viscous enough to stick to underwear. Gonorrhea produces the same type of discharge, along with a highly unpleasant odor.

Only a doctor can perform tests to determine what type of microorganism is causing the problem. Antibiotic treatments are standard procedure.

General Care

Proper hygiene is essential at all times. Wash your genitals daily and use a vaginal douche regularly.

A half-hour thyme sitz bath, once or twice a week, will stimulate circulation in the abdominal region and help your body combat harmful microorganisms. Avoid becoming overly fatigued, don't walk too much, don't go horseback riding, and abstain from sexual relations until the condition has cleared up.

Plant Power

If this is a condition that plagues you, you can use herbal remedies to supplement your doctor's care. The ones listed below have proven quite effective in helping to cure abnormal vaginal discharge.

Ladies mantle is a gynecological remedy that soothes irritation and alleviates inflammation. It is recommended for cases of uterine inflammation. Infuse 1 oz of plant in a quart of boiled water for 15 minutes (don't use metal appliances).

Elecampine is a disinfectant that helps regulate menstrual flow, and can be effective for the treatment of chronic vaginal discharge. Boil 1/2 oz of roots in a quart of water for 10 minutes; drink a couple of cups a day.

Mistletoe can be used for your daily vaginal douches. Boil 1 oz in a quart of water for a few minutes; filter, cool, and use as a douche before going to bed. Once the discharge has stopped, continue douching once a week.

White dead nettle helps cure leukorrhea (white, viscous fluid) and other types of vaginal discharge. Prepare infusions for internal use: 2/3 oz of flower tops per quart of water; drink a cup in the morning before breakfast, and two more before your main meals of the day. For hot douches, boil 1 1/2 oz of chopped plant in a quart of water for 10 minutes; filter and cool. You can also use the following mixture for douches: 1/3 oz each of white dead nettle, walnut, sage, and yarrow. Boil the mixture in a quart of water until about a cup of the water has evaporated.

Walnut is an antiseptic that helps stop abnormal vaginal discharge. Use 2/3 oz of leaves per quart of water to prepare infusions and drink two to five cups a day.

Red rose petals have a sterilizing and antibiotic effect. Prepare concentrated infusions using 1 1/2 oz to 2 oz of dried petals per quart of boiling water; cool, filter, and use as a vaginal douche.

Sage is an antiseptic that promotes healing. Drink infusions prepared with 2/3 oz of plant per quart of water.

↩ Varicose Veins

We've all seen them, and we don't want them. If we already have them, we want them even less. But what makes them happen in the first place?

As veins lose their elasticity, blood circulates less freely and tends to accumulate at a given point. Then pressure builds, causing the affected vein to weaken and become permanently dilated.

> ## BEWARE OF FAST FIXES FOR VARICOSE VEINS
>
> **D**rastic interventions like injections of sodium chloride or glucose, which actually kill a varicose vein, will not solve the problem permanently. On the contrary, they will only put a strain on the rest of your circulatory system, causing more varicose veins to appear. They can also cause thrombosis (swelling) or an embolism (sudden blocking of a blood vessel), both of which are very serious.
>
> Prevention is the best cure for varicose veins. If your legs feel heavy and red blotches appear on the skin, take immediate steps to prevent the problem from degenerating further.

A weakness in the walls of veins is often a question of heredity, but other factors can cause varicose veins to appear on the legs: cold feet, standing for long periods of time, general lack of physical movement, obesity, pregnancy, and even improper respiration. So can ingesting excessive amounts of alcohol, coffee, or tobacco.

And although we may think of varicose veins as a problem for our legs, they can pop any anywhere, including the anus (hemorrhoids), testicles and scrotum, bladder, vagina and vulva, and the pharynx and larynx. If left untreated, they can lead to complications like inflammation, varicose ulcers, and hemorrhaging.

Nutrition

Follow a hypotoxic diet. Or go on a carrot juice cure, alternating with lemon, grapefruit, or orange juice (see page 240). And avoid fats.

Vitamins C and E are essential for treating varicose veins. Vitamin C reinforces venous walls, and vitamin E tones muscles and stimulates blood circulation.

TOP TIPS FOR PREVENTING VARICOSE VEINS

- **Exercise, exercise, exercise.** It stimulates blood circulation and keeps veins open. Speed walking (about 120 steps a minute) is excellent in that it contracts and relaxes leg muscles and will improve your circulation.
- **Take a foot bath every day.** You can add 7 oz of bicarbonate of soda and 3 1/2 oz of alum to your foot baths. That will help shrink your visible veins and make you feel great in the bargain.
- **Keep your legs slightly raised when you sleep.** Place a pillow under your knees or feet. It will help keep blood from pooling in your legs.
- **Don't wear underwear or clothes that constrict your legs.** If you want to wear support stockings, put them on while sitting on a bed or chair, with your legs up in the air, after massaging the affected vein.
- **Don't wear very high heels.** They're bad for your feet and don't promote good leg circulation.
- **Avoid standing for extended periods.** Standing, especially if you're constantly in one position, will cause the blood to pool in the veins of your legs.
- **Massage.** Massage helps soothe varicose veins, but it has to be the right kind of massage: gentle rubbing and light tapping are best.

Good sources of vitamin C include green peppers and citrus fruit (oranges, grapefruit, lemons). To obtain a concentrated vitamin C extract, finely chop the peel of three lemons, two oranges, and a grapefruit and mix with some orange pulp or syrup; take two or three teaspoons a day.

Vitamin E is found in many foods, including corn and soy oil, wheat germ, and sprouted wheat.

Plant Power

Plants can help cure varicosity, notably by eliminating toxins that overload and clog your circulatory system. But don't expect miracles—although the right remedy will produce results, it may take some time.

Garlic cleans the blood, stimulates circulation, and keeps veins elastic. Soak 3 oz of peeled garlic in a quart of eau-de-vie for eight days; take a teaspoon dissolved in a glass of sweetened water every day for eight days a month. Also add garlic to soups and salads on a daily basis.

Witch hazel is an astringent and tonic that is recommended for the treatment of most types of circulation problems. You can buy the tincture in most herbal and health food stores: Take four or five drops dissolved in a little water, three times a day. You can also combine witch hazel with goldenseal: three drops of tincture of each, dissolved in a glass of water.

Ivy compresses help alleviate pain caused by varicose veins. Boil 1 1/2 oz in half a quart of water for 10 minutes.

Horse chestnuts are rich in calcium and are recommended for treating varicosity and other circulation problems. They also help alleviate pain and can be used for extended periods of time. Decoctions (1 1/2 oz per quart of water) are very bitter tasting, so you might prefer using the extract, available in herbal and health food stores, or the liqueur: Soak 1 1/2 oz of bark in a quart of white wine for one week; drink a glass before meals.

Yarrow has a tonic effect on the circulatory system and helps cure varicosity. Use 1 oz to 1 1/2 oz of flower tops per quart of water to prepare infusions and drink three or four cups a day.

Sage is recommended for external use. Boil 1 1/2 oz of sage in half a quart of water for 15 minutes and use the decoction to prepare hot compresses, or add to your foot baths.

Red grape leaves have a tonic effect on the circulatory system and are recommended for the treatment of phlebitis and varicose veins. In addition to eating red grapes, drink a cup of decoction made from the leaves before meals: Use 1 1/2 oz of leaves per quart of water.

Marigold (calendula) ointment makes an effective external treatment for varicose veins. Put two cups of flowers, leaves, and stems through a blender; mix with 1 lb of melted lard, remove from heat, and let stand for a day; filter through a fine cloth and store in sterile containers. You can also use the residue of leaves for poultices.

≫ Vomiting

For as miserable as it makes us feel, you'd think vomiting would at least have the positive attribute of pointing to some particular diagnosis, but unfortunately, it doesn't.

WHAT DO I DO IF I VOMIT BLOOD?

If you vomit blood, you should see a doctor immediately. The following symptoms can help you identify the cause of the problem, but a medical diagnosis is essential.

- **Digestive problems.** Vomiting is preceded by nausea; particles of food and gastric juices are mixed with blood; blood is red or black, depending on how long it has been in the stomach.
- **Pulmonary problems**. Blood is bright red, mixed with phlegm, and violently expelled.
- **Periodontal problems.** If blood also flows out through the nose, the problem may be hemorrhaging gums.

Vomiting of blood can also be a symptom of cirrhosis, an ulcer, an infectious disease like diphtheria or measles, a kidney stone, or even cancer.

Persons who start vomiting blood should lie down on their back, with their head slightly raised. Place an ice pack on the stomach, wrapped in some flannel or cloth. If you don't have any ice, apply a cold compress.

Don't eat solid food. You can drink clear liquid while waiting for emergency treatment, but not more than 1 1/2 quarts in a 24-hour period.

You can try adding some horsetail to liquids. It has a homeostatic effect—in other words, it stops the flow of blood. Boil 1 1/2 oz of plant in a quart of water for half an hour.

Aside from digestive problems and motion sickness, vomiting can be a symptom of many other disorders, including food poisoning, intestinal parasites, appendicitis, meningitis, or peritonitis. Vomiting is also a symptom of common childhood diseases like scarlet fever, otitis, and whooping cough. In elderly people, it can be a sign of hypertension or an impending heart attack.

Plant Power

In case of vomiting caused by indigestion, stop eating and drinking and suck on an ice cube. Hot or cold compresses can also help. Then try one of these remedies.

Aniseed is an antispasmodic that helps alleviate vomiting. Use 1/3 oz of seeds per quart of water to prepare infusions and drink two or three cups.

Lemon balm is an antispasmodic that is recommended for cases of nervousness, morning sickness, and difficult digestion. Use 1 oz per quart of water to prepare infusions, and drink three or four cups during the course of the day.

Mint is another antispasmodic and tonic recommended for cases of vomiting related to nervousness. Infuse 1 oz of dried leaves in a quart of water and drink three or four cups during the course of the day.

Linden is an antispasmodic and mild sedative recommended for cases of vomiting related to nervousness. Prepare infusions using 1 oz of leaves per quart of water and drink three or four cups a day.

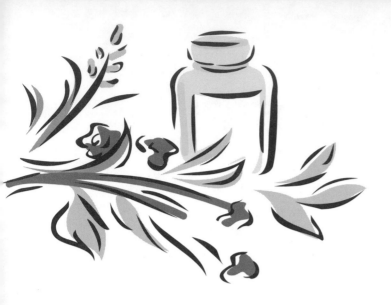

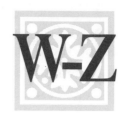

🖎 Warts

Warts may be unsightly, and you may think they belong on the backs of toads (you can't get them from toads, by the way), but with the exception of the genital variety, they present no danger to health.

Genital warts are caused by the human papilloma virus, which is transmitted through sex. They generally appear on moist areas of the genitals and anus. Women with genital warts have a higher risk for cervical cancer, and anyone having these warts in the area of the anus is more likely to get rectal cancer.

Viral warts appear mainly on the hands, feet, and face, while seborrheic warts affect mainly elderly persons. Both are harmless. How long they will last is anybody's guess. In some cases, they're life-long passengers on your body; in others, they disappear on their own.

General Care

There are various methods to remove unsightly warts: cryotherapy (freezing), electrocoagulation, radiotherapy, among others. Another method for removing warts on the hands is to burn them off by using a magnifying glass to concentrate the sun's rays—repeat on a number of consecutive days.

Plant Power

Plants can also be effective for removing viral and seborrheic warts. Apply one of the remedies listed below every second day, and lightly rub the wart you want to remove with a pumice stone. For genital warts, see a doctor.

Garlic can be used to treat warts in winter, when plants like celandine and marigold are not available. Prepare an ointment by peeling and grating three large cloves of garlic and adding a little olive oil; apply twice a day. At night apply garlic poultices (make sure to protect the surrounding skin with a bandage).

Celandine is very effective for removing warts. The treatment usually takes about eight days. Simply apply fresh celandine juice twice a day: Snap a stem of the plant and squeeze the sap right onto the wart (do not spread on surrounding skin). Continue the treatment for eight days to two weeks, after which the wart should fall off. Do not put any sap in your mouth, because this plant is poisonous.

Marigold has the same effect as celandine. Use it in the same way—apply fresh sap twice a day for eight days to two weeks.

≈ Water Retention

One day your favorite ring fits you, the next day you can't get it over your finger. Or you wake up in the morning and the shoes you've worn for the past six months suddenly feel so tight that your feet can't stand them. It's all due to water retention, also called edema, which makes the tissues of your body swell up. Swelling can occur under the skin; in mucous membranes in the nose, throat, larynx or genitals; in the lungs (acute pulmonary edema); and on the face (Quincke's edema).

The remedies in this section concern only benign cases. Acute pulmonary edema, which can bring about extreme shortness of breath, anxiety, and copious amounts of orange mucous in the lungs, requires immediate emergency care.

Quincke's edema can also be life threatening if it affects the larynx and blocks the respiratory passages.

Determining the Cause

In order to determine what's causing your swelling, look for the following symptoms:

- Edema that first affects the eyelids is caused by a kidney malfunction.
- Edema the starts in the abdominal region is caused by a liver problem.
- Edema first appearing in the lower limbs is caused by a heart problem.

Plant Power

If you have generalized swelling with hives, adopt a hypotoxic diet (see Appendix B), avoid salt, and don't drink a lot (ideally less than the amount you urinate). Make sure you are getting a full range of vitamins. Then try some of these remedies.

Wild garlic helps clean out the kidneys and bladder and facilitates evacuation. It is especially recommended for elderly persons. Take 10 to 15 drops of garlic liqueur, four times a day: Fill a container with fresh chopped leaves (don't press) or finely chopped cloves; cover with 40-proof alcohol, and let stand in direct sunlight or near some other heat source for 15 days.

Birch is a diuretic that is effective for treating edema. Prepare infusions using 1 oz to 2 oz of leaves per quart of water and drink three to five cups a day, between meals.

Cherry is a powerful diuretic. Soak 5 oz of dried cherry stems in a quart of water; boil for a quarter of an hour, then remove from heat and let stand for 10 minutes. You can also add 1 oz of bearberry (uva ursi) leaves or some slices of apple to tastc; filter, and sip throughout the day.

Common broom is another diuretic recommended for cases of edema. The plant stimulates the elimination of large amounts of urine, giving the kidneys a chance to recover. Common broom also acts as a heart tonic, regulating circulation and curing another possible cause of edema. Add 1 oz to 2 oz of dried flowers to a quart of cold water, boil for two or three minutes, filter, and sweeten with honey. Drink three lukewarm cups a day, between meals.

Queen of the meadow is recommended for edema of the lower limbs, because it helps drain liquid from tissues. Add 1 oz of flower tops to a quart of water at not more than 175 degrees Fahrenheit (a higher temperature will destroy the plant's active ingredient—salicylate), and let stand for a few minutes. Drink two or three cups a day.

Note: Do not use this remedy if you're allergic to aspirin or ibuprophen.

Elder combats inflammation linked to kidney problems and thus alleviates edema. Boil 1/2 oz of elder in 10 oz of water until half the water has evaporated; drink two half-cups during the course of the day.

➽ Weight (Too Low)

If you have always been skinny but feel comfortable and suffer from no unusual health problems, then enjoy your good luck.

If, however, you suddenly start losing weight because you have been sick or because of improper nutrition, then there's lots you can do to help stimulate your appetite and regain those lost pounds.

Nutrition

The idea is not to stuff yourself with food but to gradually regain your appetite. Your diet should be varied and rich in vitamins, especially vitamins B1, B2, C, and D. Add wheat germ, which is full of essential nutrients and helps tone your nervous system, to salads, soups, and cereals. You can also obtain wheat germ powder, which you can mix with a little milk or water and drink before meals—one tablespoon for adults and one teaspoon for children.

Eat a lot of fruit and vegetables (celery, chicory, cabbage, watercress, spinach, carrots, turnips, red cabbage, lentils). Also recommended are eggs, red meat, and calves liver.

Brewer's yeast is another food supplement that is just bursting with nutrients. If you think you might have developed a nutritional deficiency, add a tablespoon of brewer's yeast (a teaspoon for children) to soups, stews, breakfast cereals, etc.

Plant Power

Herbs can be great appetite stimulators if you know which ones to use. Try these. You'll be pleased with the results.

ANOREXIA

Anorexia nervosa is an eating disorder that can kill you. People who suffer with it—mostly young women—become so obsessed with losing weight that they begin to starve themselves. The tremendous stress this places on the body can eventually become deadly.

Anorexics are typically more than 15 percent below normal body weight, are obsessed with food and weight, often exercise too much, and may even participate in strange eating rituals. Women with this disorder often stop menstruating.

Anorexia is thought to be the result of pressure—whether real or imagined—to live up to some standard of beauty imposed by society. The condition can also be caused by deep-seated psychological problems.

If you or someone in your family is suffering from anorexia, you must absolutely seek the help of a doctor or qualified psychotherapist. And be prepared to get the entire family involved. Anorexics need the support of everyone around them as they begin to heal, so it's not uncommon for psychologists to ask family members to participate in treatment programs.

There is no point in trying to impose medications—including plant remedies—until the underlying psychological causes of the problem are addressed.

Angelica is known to have a beneficial effect on the kidneys and to stimulate appetite. Prepare infusions using 2/3 oz of leaves per cup of water, let stand for 10 to 15 minutes, filter, and drink.

Fenugreek has such a pronounced effect that you should take it only for one or two weeks at a time. Mix a teaspoon of powdered seeds with an equal amount of honey. Take one teaspoon morning and night.

Sweet flag also stimulates appetite and facilitates the elimination of waste. Prepare infusions using the roots, which you soak overnight in a cup of cold water. Reheat slightly in a double steamer, then filter and drink. You can also add this plant to your bath water: Soak 1 lb of roots in five quarts of water overnight; next morning bring to a boil and add to your bath water.

Weight (Too High)

"I just need to take off ten or fifteen pounds . . ."

How many times have you heard someone say that? A lot

of people daydream about losing weight without making any effort at all. And no wonder, what with all the miracle diets and exercise gadgets you see advertised these days.

Unfortunately, there is a simple reason why so many people are over-weight—they eat too much. And if there is one thing that is difficult to change, it is a habit, like overeating, that is deeply ingrained.

The question is: Is this habit worth changing? There are, as everyone knows, health risks associated with obesity, but recent research shows that you can be both overweight and healthy if you exercise properly.

So ask yourself why you want to lose those 10 or 15 pounds. Is it out of a desire to be loved?

If you dislike yourself because you're a few pounds heavier than you should be, then getting rid of those excess pounds might very well solve your problem. On the other hand, getting rid of one problem may simply cause another to arise. In other words, if your self-esteem problems go deeper than your fat levels, you'll just find another reason to dislike yourself, once you've reached your weight-loss goal.

So remember, as you're deciding whether to embark on a weight-loss plan, that what is important is how you feel about yourself. Real beauty is the result of being satisfied with the way you look, even if you're a few pounds overweight.

You should also be aware that the faster you lose weight, the faster you tend to gain it back. The only way to really benefit from a weight-loss program is to make permanent changes to your eating habits and maintain those changes even after you've lost weight. You may have to avoid certain foods and cut others out of your diet altogether.

Nutrition

There are two key factors for controlling your weight: eating a healthy, balanced diet and getting enough exercise. Not only will these measures help combat a weight problem, they will also reduce your stress level, fight disease, and contribute to your overall sense of well being.

Start off by taking fats and white sugar out of your daily diet. Pineapples, celery, and tomatoes are three delicious foods that can be used to replace them without depriving your taste buds of the pleasures they crave.

NATURE'S OWN WEIGHT-LOSS ELIXIR

Here's an herbal elixir that's great for weight loss. Combine the following plants and infuse in a quart of water:

1 pinch of hyssop
1 pinch of rosemary
1/3 oz of dog's tooth
1/3 oz of buckthorn
1 oz of red grape leaves

Drink a cup before meals, morning and evening.

Plant Power

Plants can help you lose weight in many ways. Some promote better elimination of waste, some purify your blood, while others facilitate digestion. Here are the best ones to try.

Irish moss and carob can be taken in gel cap form an hour before meals to make you feel full and thereby reduce the amount of food you eat at each sitting.

Ash is a powerful diuretic that will make any weight loss diet you are on more effective. Prepare infusions using ash leaves and drink on a regular basis.

Horehound is reputed to be helpful for losing weight. Use 2/3 oz per quart of water when preparing your infusions and drink three or four cups a day.

Maté acts as a stimulant, diuretic, and antiseptic. When taken as an infusion, it helps fight the sensation of hunger.

❧ Whooping Cough

Whooping cough (pertussis) is a childhood disease that can have serious consequences in young infants. Despite vaccinations that inhibit its development, the disease can still be transmitted through direct contact.

The incubation period lasts about eight days, followed by initial symptoms that resemble those of a common cold: runny nose, slight fever (about 100 degrees Fahrenheit), and dry coughing, especially at night.

It is the dry coughing that is most characteristic of the disorder. Children become anxious as their small bodies are wracked by coughing spasms that can stop them momentarily from breathing (some children experience up to 100 such coughing fits a day) and leave them gasping for air. Infants suffering from whooping cough quickly become exhausted and tend to turn blue during coughing fits, which causes them to vomit.

General Care

Affected children should be isolated and kept in a well-ventilated room. There's no need to keep them in bed unless they are running a high fever or develop other complications. A doctor will invariably prescribe antibiotics. You can use natural

> ## NATURAL COUGH MEDICINE FOR WHOOPING COUGH
>
> **W**hooping cough can be as frightening for parents as it is for the kids who get it. But with a little help from this herbal elixir, both you and your child can get a better night's sleep.
>
> You'll need the help of an herbalist or pharmacist. Ask him or her to combine sundew and red poppy as a syrup: 2 grams of sundew tincture in 200 grams of red poppy syrup.

remedies to alleviate coughing and build resistance. Administering a diuretic will help the kidneys eliminate toxins.

Nutrition

Food should be easy to swallow, composed of purées and creams, and finely chopped or minced meat, served in small portions at regular intervals.

Plant Power

Here are some plants that can help kids get through the rough spots, but don't give anything to infants without your doctor's approval.

Mullein helps stop bronchial secretions, alleviates coughing, and soothes chest inflammation. Give children a cup of infusion between meals and one before going to bed at night. To prepare infusions, use 1 oz of flowers per quart of boiling water; remove from heat and let stand for 10 minutes; filter through a fine cloth (linen or cotton).

Eucalyptus is a bronchial antiseptic and expectorant that helps control coughing fits. The plant also acts as a general stimulant. Serve children four cups of infusion per day. To prepare infusions, use 1 oz of leaves per quart of water; remove from heat and let stand for 30 minutes. You can also steam eucalyptus to prepare an antiseptic and antibacterial vapor: Add 1/3 oz of essence of eucalyptus to a quart of boiling water, or boil a handful of leaves in the sickroom, leaving the pot uncovered.

Lavender is a diuretic that soothes bronchial irritation, alleviates spasms, and acts as a pulmonary antiseptic. Prepare decoctions by boiling 2/3 oz of lavender in a quart of water for five minutes; remove from heat, and let stand for 10 minutes.

Milkwort is an expectorant that combats persistent coughing and stimulates perspiration, which eliminates toxins. Serve children four teaspoons of infusion a day. To prepare infusions, use 1/3 oz per 3 oz of boiling water; remove from heat, and let stand for five minutes.

Horseradish poultices help dissolve pulmonary congestion. Use freshly grated horseradish and limit applications to 15 to 20 minutes (less for delicate skin).

Thyme helps alleviate anxiety. It also reduces bronchial secretions and inhibits spasms caused by convulsive dry coughing. Prepare a thyme-based syrup by adding 7 oz of honey to 3 oz of hot thyme infusion (1 pinch per 3 oz of boiling water). You can also combine thyme with plantain, which has a soothing effect, alleviates coughing, and facilitates expectoration. To prepare infusions, use a pinch of thyme and a pinch of plantain per 3 oz of boiling water. Give children four or five cups a day of the freshly prepared infusion or a mouthful every hour to reduce the risk of pulmonary inflammation.

PART III

The Fundamentals of Foods and Herbs

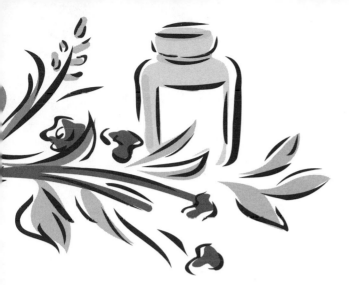

Medicinal Plants A-Z

This alphabetical listing allows you to locate any of the plants listed in the encyclopedia, and provides you with instant information about their various applications.

Absinthe
Facilitates digestion, accelerates healing. Recommended for the treatment of colic, hiccups, and loss of appetite.

Agrimony
Astringent, promotes bile secretions. Recommended for the treatment of angina, diarrhea, digestive problems, liver problems, sore throat, gallstones, jaundice.

Alder
Recommended for the treatment of anemia, asthenia, liver problems, infection, leucorrhea, appetite loss.

Algae
Promotes longevity.

Alkegenge
Absorbs excess acid, diuretic. Recommended for the treatment of rheumatism.

Almond
Alleviates inflammation. Recommended for the treatment of stomach and duodenal ulcers, skin eruptions.

Aloe Vera
Laxative, accelerates healing of burns, alleviates inflammation. Recommended for the treatment of arthritis, minor cuts and wounds, burns, cancer, colitis, constipation, chapped skin, skin cancer.

Angelica
Facilitates digestion, regulates menstruation, reduces fever, acts as a sedative. Recommended for the treatment of asthenia, bronchitis, convalescence, fever, hiccups, indigestion, lack of appetite, memory loss, cuts and wounds, pneumonia, difficult menstruation, cough.

Aniseed
Facilitates digestion. Recommended for the treatment of colic, appetite loss, halitosis, aerophagia.

Apple
Recommended for the treatment of hypertension.

Arnica
Hypotensive. Recommended for the treatment of minor injuries, sprains, hypertension, stiff neck.

Artichoke
Tonic, remineralizes the body. Recommended for the treatment of acne, arthritis, atherosclerosis, cholecystitis, high cholesterol, cirrhosis, liver attacks and liver problems, jaundice, gallstones.

Ash
Astringent. Recommended for the treatment of obesity, fever, gout, urinary infections.

Barberry (Berberis)
Recommended for the treatment of venous problems.

Barley
Recommended for the treatment of psoriasis and other skin problems, wrinkles.

Basil
Recommended for the treatment of anxiety.

Bearberry (Uva Ursi)
Recommended for the treatment of prostate problems, urethritis, urinary disorders.

Bedstraw
Recommended for the treatment of cancer, acne, and blackheads.

Beet
Recommended for the treatment of vitiligo.

Birch
Recommended for the treatment of abscesses, albuminuria, cellulite, high cholesterol, hepatic colic, gout, impetigo, edema, rheumatism, seborrhea, excessive perspiration, urticaria.

Bistort
Recommended for the treatment of diarrhea, gingivitis, stomatitis.

Bitter Milkwort
Recommended for the treatment of whooping cough, pulmonary catarrh, laryngitis.

Bittersweet
Recommended for the treatment of high cholesterol, dermatitis.

Bladderwrack
Recommended for the treatment of obesity.

Blackberry
Recommended for the treatment of diabetes, angina, diarrhea, dysentery.

Blackcurrant
Recommended for the treatment of diarrhea, insect bites, senility.

Black Hemp Nettle
Recommended for the treatment of obesity, asthma, bronchitis, appetite loss, tuberculosis and other pulmonary disorders.

Black Radish
Recommended for the treatment of cholecystitis, boils, gallstones.

Blueberry
Recommended for the treatment of conjunctivitis, ophthalmia, senility.

Boldo
Recommended for the treatment of liver and uterine problems.

Borage
Recommended for the treatment of abscesses, urinary problems, bronchitis, lupus, nephritis, pneumonia, head colds, measles, cough, urethritis.

Broom Heather
Recommended for the treatment of cellulite, colibacillosis, acute urinary disorders, cystitis, prostate problems, chest angina, ringing in the ears, uremia.

Buckbean (Bogbean)
Recommended for the treatment of anemia and fever.

Buckthorn
Recommended for the treatment of constipation.

Buckwheat
Promotes longevity. Recommended for the treatment of hypertension.

Burdock
Recommended for the treatment of abscesses, acne, tonsillitis, arthritis, dull dry hair, dermatitis, diabetes, boils, gout, herpes, impetigo, pruritis, psoriasis, pyorrhea, rheumatism, seborrhea, complexion problems, ulcers, hives, eye problems.

Butterburr
Antibiotic. Recommended for the treatment of asthma, cuts and wounds, cancer.

Cabbage
Recommended for the treatment of abscesses, acne, angina, boils, impetigo, cuts and wounds, pruritis, rheumatism, sciatica, tumors, varicose ulcers, stomach and duodenal ulcers.

Caraway

Aperitif and carminative; stimulates milk production in breast-feeding mothers. Recommended for the treatment of aerophagia, digestive problems, lack of appetite.

Cardamom

Recommended for the treatment of digestive problems, halitosis.

Carob

Recommended for the treatment of diarrhea.

Carrot

Remineralizes the body—depurative. Recommended for the treatment of anemia, diarrhea, burns, dermatitis, digestive problems, impetigo, skin problems.

Catnip

Recommended for the treatment of dysmenorrhea.

Cayenne

Recommended for the treatment of sore throat.

Celandine

Recommended for the treatment of dermatitis, chest angina, cancer, skin cancer, acne and blackheads, corns (on the feet), liver problems, jaundice, ophthalmia, cholecystitis, cataracts, psoriasis, eye problems.

Celery

Aperitif, carminative, depurative, choleretic. Recommended for the treatment of acne, obesity, gout.

Centaury

Aperitif. Recommended for the treatment of appetite loss, burnout, distended stomach, liver problems, anemia, fever, urticaria.

Chamomile

Antispasmodic, facilitates digestion, sedative, accelerates healing. Recommended for the treatment of blisters, arthritis, dull dry hair, colic, conjunctivitis, digestive problems, dysmenorrhea, nervousness, fever, chapped skin, insomnia, appetite loss, migraines, nausea, morning sickness, neuralgia, ophthalmia, intestinal parasites, difficult menstruation, rheumatism, head colds, sinusitis, stress, minor injuries, eye problems, headaches, inflammation.

Cherry

Recommended for the treatment of obesity, edema, uremia, gout.

Chervil

Depurative, digestive. Recommended for the treatment of digestive problems, ophthalmia.

Chickweed

Recommended for the treatment of convulsions.

Chicory

Choleretic, cholagogic, depurative, laxative tonic, remineralizes the body. Recommended for the treatment of constipation, dermatitis, diabetes, liver problems, hyperglycemia, jaundice, gallstones, heart problems, hepatic colic, obesity.

Chinchona

Recommended for the treatment of fever.

Cinnamon

Recommended for the treatment of the flu.

Clove

Recommended for the treatment of depression, neuralgia, dental pain.

Club Moss

Recommended for the treatment of cancer, scars, sty.

Coltsfoot

Expectorant. Recommended for the treatment of blisters, asthma, bronchitis, phlebitis, foot problems, head colds, cough, ulcers.

Comfrey

Recommended for the treatment of arthritis, cuts and wounds, burns, cancer, gout, skin problems, menstrual problems, rheumatism, wrinkles, stiff neck, ulcers, varicosity.

Common Broom
Recommended for the treatment of liver problems, jaundice, cuts and wounds, pneumonia, edema.

Coriander
Carminative, digestive. Recommended for the treatment of depression, digestive problems, memory loss.

Corn
Recommended for the treatment of arthritis, rheumatism, obesity.

Couchgrass (Doggrass)
Cholagogic, depurative, laxative. Recommended for the treatment of colic, liver problems, acne, constipation, dermatitis, flu, jaundice, gallstones, uremia.

Cow Parsnip
Recommended for the treatment of abscesses, frigidity, ulcers.

Cucumber
Recommended for the treatment of skin problems and wrinkles.

Cumin
Carminative, digestive. Recommended for the treatment of digestive problems, halitosis. Stimulates milk production in breast-feeding mothers.

Cypress
Astringent. Recommended for the treatment of vitiligo, menopausal problems.

Daisy
Stimulant. Recommended for the treatment of skin spots.

Damiania
Aphrodisiac. Recommended during periods of convalescence.

Dandelion
Depurative, antiseptic, cholagogic. Recommended for the treatment of high cholesterol, dermatitis, diabetes, liver problems, boils, hyperglycemia, jaundice, gallstones, pruritis, rheumatism, stress, urinary infections.

Depurative Remedy

Recommended for the treatment of arthritis, cancer, cataracts, scars, digestive problems, fever, liver problems, gout, inflammation, appetite loss, rheumatism, measles, complexion problems, tumors.

Devil's Claw

Recommended for the treatment of rheumatism.

Digitalis

Heart tonic. Recommended for the treatment of infarct, tachycardia, palpitations.

Dill

Expels gas from the stomach and intestines, acts as a general stimulant. Recommended for the treatment of vomiting and halitosis.

Eggplant

Has a sedative, relaxing effect.

Elder

Emollient, sudorific. Recommended for the treatment of nephritis, edema, ophthalmia, sty, rheumatism, stomatitis.

Eucalyptus

Antiseptic, disinfectant, expectorant, sedative, heart tonic. Recommended for the treatment of urinary infections, bronchitis, cuts and wounds, cystitis, whooping cough, diabetes, digestive problems, fever, hyperglycemia, head colds, sinusitis, urethritis, cough.

Eyebright

Recommended for the treatment of eye problems, ophthalmia, head colds.

Fennel

Carminative, stimulates milk production in breast-feeding mothers, general stimulant. Recommended for the treatment of aerophagia, flu, rheumatism, breast problems, urinary infections.

Fenugreek

Recommended for the treatment of obesity, anemia, boils, hyperglycemia, sinusitis, tuberculosis and other pulmonary disorders.

Fir Balsam
Recommended for the treatment of head colds.

Fumitory
General tonic. Recommended for the treatment of dermatitis, herpes, urticaria.

Galanga
Recommended for the treatment of rheumatism.

Garlic
Antiseptic, antibiotic, heart tonic, hypotensive. Recommended for the treatment of asthma, atherosclerosis, infarct, palpitations, tachycardia, corns on the feet, cystitis, dental problems, hypertension, infections, infectious diseases, intestinal parasites, phlebitis, rheumatism, measles, varicosity, venous problems, arteriosclerosis, diarrhea, edema, warts.

Gentian
Aperitif, cholagogic, depurative, heart tonic. Recommended for the treatment of anemia, digestive problems, fever, liver problems, appetite loss, intestinal parasites.

Geranium
Recommended for the treatment of stomach and duodenal ulcers.

Ginger
Aphrodisiac. Recommended for the treatment of dysmenorrhea, sprains.

Ginseng
General tonic, aphrodisiac, promotes longevity. Recommended for the treatment of fatigue, burnout, acne, asthenia, appetite loss, memory loss, and for use during periods of convalescence.

Goat's Rue
Recommended for the treatment of diabetes, hyperglycemia, breast problems.

Goldenrod
Antiseptic. Recommended for the treatment of urinary infections, cellulite, cystitis, hay fever, urethritis, gout.

Goldenseal
Antiseptic. Recommended for the treatment of urinary disorders and other types of infection, cystitis, prostatitis, hay fever, cuts and wounds.

Gotu Kola
Promotes longevity. Recommended for the treatment of memory loss.

Grapes
Recommended for the treatment of obesity.

Hawthorn
Recommended for the treatment of chest angina, anxiety, arrhythmia, atherosclerosis, ringing in the ears, infarct, palpitations, tachycardia, depression, hypertension, hysteria, insomnia, menopausal problems, nervousness, burnout, vertigo.

Hedge Mustard
Recommended for the treatment of laryngitis, tobacco addiction.

Hops
Anaphrodisiac, aperitif, sedative, depurative, stimulates milk production in breast-feeding women. Recommended for the treatment of anemia, sexual excitation, insomnia, appetite loss, nervousness, stomach and duodenal ulcers.

Horehound (White)
Heart tonic, expectorant. Recommended for the treatment of arrhythmia, infarct, palpitations, tachycardia, fever.

Horse Chestnut
Recommended for the treatment of varicosity.

Horseradish
Antibiotic. Recommended for the treatment of anemia, angina, scurvy, whooping cough, rheumatism, skin spots.

Horsetail
Depurative, antiseptic, homeostatic. Recommended for the treatment of albuminarea, blisters, bronchitis, cancer, glaucoma, hemorrhage, hemorrhoids, lupus, difficult menstruation, nephritis, nosebleed, engorged breasts, pulmonary tuberculosis, tumors, ulcers, vomiting blood.

Houseleek
Recommended for the treatment of various zonae.

Hyssop
Recommended for the treatment of angina, asthma.

Icelandic Moss
Recommended for the treatment of vomiting.

Irish Moss (Carageen)
Recommended for persons trying to lose weight.

Ivy
Recommended for the treatment of asthma, cellulite, varicosity, venous problems, bronchitis, catarrh, pulmonary disorders including tuberculosis, head colds, hay fever, cough.

Juniper
Depurative, antiseptic, stimulant. Recommended for the treatment of urethritis.

Kelp
Promotes longevity. Cures an iodine deficiency.

Knotgrass
Recommended for the treatment of incontinence, pulmonary tuberculosis.

Lapacho
Recommended for the treatment of cancer.

Lavender
Antiseptic, decongestant, choleretic, sedative. Recommended for the treatment of anxiety, asthma, whooping cough, bronchitis, depression, nervousness, flu, migraines, intestinal parasites, insect bites, cough, ulcers, vertigo.

Leek
Recommended for the treatment of dull hair, skin fissures.

Lemon
Recommended for the treatment of halitosis, wrinkles, venous problems, eye problems, flu, mineral or vitamin deficiencies.

Lemon Balm (Melissa)

Antispasmodic, sedative, carminative, digestive, expectorant, relaxant, heart tonic. Recommended for the treatment of anxiety, depression, digestive problems, memory loss, nervousness, neurasthenia, palpitations, difficult menstruation, syncope, vertigo.

Lettuce

Sedative, anaphrodisiac, antispasmodic, relaxant.

Licorice

Recommended for the treatment of colitis, laryngitis, stomach and duodenal ulcers.

Lily

Recommended for the treatment of acne rosacea (couperose), skin spots.

Lily of the Valley

Heart tonic. Recommended for the treatment of infarct, palpitations, tachycardia, headaches, sinusitis.

Linden

Relaxant, antispasmodic, sedative. Recommended for the treatment of anxiety, arthritis, atherosclerosis, hepatic colic, aches and pains, depression, flu, hypertension, sunburn, insomnia, migraines, nervousness, sciatica, venous problems, vomiting.

Linseed

Emollient, laxative. Recommended for the treatment of constipation, inflammation, gallstones, infectious diseases.

Lotus

Recommended for the treatment of insomnia.

Maidenhair

Recommended for the treatment of coughs.

Malva

Emollient, antiseptic. Recommended for the treatment of abscesses, tonsillitis, colic, dermatitis, herpes, inflammation, orchitis, skin problems, pruritis, head colds, wrinkles, stomach and duodenal ulcers.

Marigold

Cholagogic, homeostatic. Recommended for the treatment of blisters, burns, cancer, dermatitis, liver problems, sprains, scabies, glaucoma, hematuria, hemorrhage, jaundice, impetigo, inflammation, skin cancer, phlebitis, foot problems, pneumonia, difficult menstruation, skin spots, tumors, ulcers, varicosity, warts.

Marjoram

Recommended for the treatment of cancer, sore throat, nervousness.

Marshmallow

Emollient, mild sedative. Recommended for the treatment of abscesses, angina, arthritis, bronchitis, colic, infant teething, dermatitis, pruritis, cough.

Maté

Heart tonic, stimulant. Recommended for the treatment of obesity, infarct, palpitations, tachycardia, neurasthenia, burnout.

Melilot (Sweet Clover)

Antispasmodic.

Milk (Carline) Thistle

Recommended for the treatment of neurasthenia.

Millet

Recommended for the treatment of arthritis.

Mint

Antiseptic, carminative, expectorant, sudorific. Recommended for the treatment of dental problems, depression, dermatitis, frigidity, halitosis, hiccups, menopausal problems, migraines, skin problems, engorged breasts, vertigo, vomiting.

Mistletoe

Antiseptic, tonic. Recommended for the treatment of fatigue, burnout, atherosclerosis, cancer, heart problems, infarct, palpitations, tachycardia, nervousness, dysentery, hypertension, hypotension, hysteria, menopausal problems, vertigo.

Mountain Wormwood
Facilitates digestion.

Mullein
Recommended for the treatment of asthma, bronchitis, burns, whooping cough, flu, hemorrhoids, inflammation, intestinal parasites, cuts and wounds, cough, tuberculosis.

Mustard
Recommended for the treatment of arthritis, bronchitis, pneumonia.

Myrtle
Antiseptic. Recommended for the treatment of diarrhea, urinary infections, cystitis, diabetes, dysentery, hyperglycemia, stomatitis.

Nasturtium
Antibiotic, aphrodisiac. Recommended for the treatment of hair loss (alopecia), senility.

Nettle
Depurative, homeostatic. Recommended for the treatment of hair loss, anemia, angina, cancer, dermatitis, diabetes, digestive problems, boils, hemorrhage, hypertension, hyperglycemia, metrorrhagia, rheumatism, sciatica, stress, complexion problems, pulmonary tuberculosis, tumors, urticaria.

Oak
Recommended for the treatment of anemia, hemorrhoids.

Oats
Stimulant and tonic, remineralizes the body. Recommended for the treatment of dry cracked skin.

Olive
Choleretic (stimulates bile secretions), antiseptic. Recommended for the treatment of fever, hypertension, hypotension, nails, skin and hair.

Onion
Recommended for the treatment of albuminurea, hair loss, dull hair, sprains, boils, intestinal parasites, insect bites, head colds, measles, sinusitis, urinary disorders.

Orange
Antispasmodic, sedative. Recommended for the treatment of anxiety, fever, insomnia, migraines, nervousness.

Oregano
Aromatic.

Ortosiphon
Recommended for the treatment of uremia.

Pansy
Depurative. Recommended for the treatment of acne, dermatitis, psoriasis, gout, rheumatism.

Papaya
Recommended for the treatment of infections.

Parsley
Carminative, depurative, promotes longevity. Recommended for the treatment of difficult menstruation, fever, insect bites, rickets, rheumatism, engorged breasts.

Passion Flower
Antispasmodic, relaxant. Recommended for the treatment of insomnia.

Pellitory-of-the-Wall
Recommended for the treatment of hemorrhoids, prostate problems.

Peppermint
Recommended for the treatment of digestive problems.

Pimpernel
Stimulates milk production in pregnant mothers.

Pine
Antiseptic, disinfectant, expectorant. Recommended for the treatment of respiratory disorders, sinusitis, urethritis and other urinary infections, prostate problems.

Plantain
Recommended for the treatment of diarrhea, cuts and wounds, catarrh, conjunctivitis, infant teething, dermatitis, infectious diseases, ophthalmia, insect bites, tuberculosis, tumors, ulcers.

Pollen
Food supplement. Recommended during periods of convalescence.

Poplar
Recommended for the treatment of venous problems.

Poppy (Red)
Recommended for the treatment of coughs and whooping cough.

Poppy Seeds
Recommended for the treatment of wrinkles.

Primrose (Cowslip)
Recommended for the treatment of rheumatism.

Pumpkin Seeds
Recommended for the treatment of intestinal parasites.

Purple Loosestrife
Recommended for the treatment of difficult menstruation, pruritis.

Queen of the Meadow
Antiseptic, astringent, sudorific. Recommended for the treatment of obesity, urinary infections, arthritis, cellulite, digestive problems, neuralgia, edema, rheumatism, sciatica, stomach and duodenal ulcers.

Radish
Stimulates bile secretions. Recommended for the treatment of liver problems.

Red Grape Leaves
Recommended for the treatment of obesity, menopausal problems, venous problems.

Restharrow
Recommended for the treatment of obesity.

Rhubarb
Recommended for the treatment of digestive problems.

Rose
Astringent. Recommended for the treatment of infections, inflammation, leucorrhea, ophthalmia, skin problems, wrinkles, eye problems, sore throat, angina, tuberculosis.

Rosemary

Cholagogic, decongestant. Recommended for the treatment of hair loss, asthenia, high cholesterol, fever, liver problems, frigidity, flu, memory loss, palpitations, liver problems, skin problems, burnout, cough, physical injuries.

Rue

Recommended for the treatment of eye problems.

Rye (Ergot)

Recommended for the treatment of migraines.

Saffron

Aromatic.

Sage

Antiseptic, aperitif, carminative, aromatic, antisudorific. Recommended for the treatment of acne, tonsillitis, dull dry hair, dental problems, depression, digestive problems, fever, liver problems, frigidity, gum disorders, sore throat, halitosis, impetigo, infections, inflammation, leucorrhea, appetite loss, menopausal problems, skin problems, insect bites, psoriasis, pyorrhea, difficult menstruation, rheumatism, measles, sterility, burnout, excessive perspiration, tuberculosis, varicosity, varicose ulcers, vertigo.

Sarsaparilla

Recommended for the treatment of dermatitis, sterility.

Sesame

Promotes longevity.

Shepherd's Purse

Recommended for the treatment of albuminuria, dysmenorrhea, hemorrhaging, low blood pressure, difficult menstruation, urethritis, varicosity.

Silverweed

Recommended for the treatment of leucorrhea, ulcers.

Soapwort

Recommended for the treatment of various zonae.

Sorrel

Recommended for the treatment of tumors.

Speedwell
Recommended for the treatment of high cholesterol, liver problems, glaucoma, pruritis, burnout, cough, nervousness.

Spinach
Remineralizes the body.

St. John's wort
Antiseptic. Recommended for the treatment of urinary infections, cuts and burns, cystitis, hysteria, sprains and bruises, neuralgia, rheumatism, sciatica, injuries of all kinds, tumors.

Star Anis
Recommended for the treatment of halitosis.

Strawberry
Antiseptic. Recommended for the treatment of wrinkles, intestinal problems, dysentery.

Sundew
Recommended for the treatment of whooping cough.

Sunflower Seeds
Promote longevity.

Sweet Flag
Recommended for the treatment of gastric acidity, obesity, cancer, digestive problems, foot problems, tobacco addiction.

Sweet Woodruff
Recommended for the treatment of liver problems, insomnia, stress.

Tarragon
Recommended for the treatment of digestive and menstrual problems.

Thistle
Recommended for the treatment of phlebitis, anemia, low blood pressure.

Thyme
Aromatic, carminative, choleretic, depurative, digestive. Recommended for the treatment of asthenia, colitis, whooping cough, dental problems, depression, digestive problems, difficult menstruation, gingivitis, sore throat, flu,

infections, leucorrhea, migraines, nervousness, neurasthenia, intestinal parasites, rickets, skin problems, head colds, measles, sinusitis, tumors, burnout, ulcers, uremia, urinary infections.

Tomato
Recommended for the treatment of acne.

Valerian
Sedative. Recommended for the treatment of anxiety, asthma, convulsions, depression, nervousness, sexual excitation, insomnia, neurasthenia, palpitations, tetanus.

Verbena
Sedative, relaxant. Recommended for the treatment of digestive problems, frigidity, insomnia, neuralgia, stress, rheumatism, and during periods of convalescence.

Violet
Recommended for the treatment of psoriasis.

Walnut
Astringent, depurative. Recommended for the treatment of albuminurea, hair loss, angina, conjunctivitis, dermatitis, diabetes, gingivitis, scabies, sore throat, hyperglycemia, impetigo, pyorrhea, rickets, tumors, varicose ulcers, ulcers.

Watercress
Expectorant, depurative. Recommended for the treatment of acne, hair loss, scurvy, dental problems, dermatitis, rheumatism, tobacco addiction.

Water Lily
Recommended for the treatment of sexual excitation, tetanus.

Wheat Germ
Food supplement, especially recommended during periods of convalescence.

White Bryony
Recommended for the treatment of sciatica.

White Dead Nettle
Recommended for the treatment of leucorrhea, metrorrhagia, orchitis.

Wild Thyme

Astringent, aromatic, digestive, carminative. Recommended for the treatment of digestive problems, intestinal parasites, cough.

Windflower

Relaxant. Recommended for the treatment of headaches.

Witch Hazel

Recommended for the treatment of hemorrhoids, varicosity, venous problems.

Wormwood

Facilitates digestion. Recommended for the treatment of gangrene, difficult menstruation, nervousness.

Yarrow

Antiseptic, heart tonic, sedative, stimulates menstrual flow, reduces fever, promotes coagulation of blood. Recommended for the treatment of cancer, fever, hemorrhage, hemorrhoids, pyorrhea, leucorrhea, nose bleed, rickets, irregular menstruation, breast problems and tumors, menopausal problems, phlebitis, varicosity, venous problems.

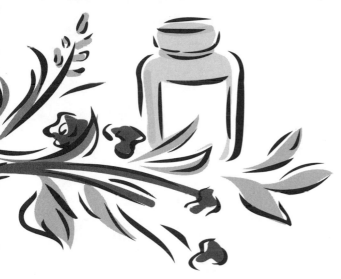

Vitamins and Minerals A-Z

You already know that vitamins and minerals are indispensable for health, but if you want to get their full benefit, there are some rules to follow.

• When you get home after shopping for food, put your vegetables in the fridge or pantry right away: some vitamins (A, B1, B2, B6, D, K, L1, L2) are destroyed by exposure to light.

• Cooking vegetables for too long destroys much of their vitamin content. Vitamins A, B1, B5, C, and D are very sensitive to heat. It's best to steam vegetables or use only a little boiling water in a covered pan, for a short time. The crunchier a vegetable is, the better it tastes and the richer it is in nutrients.

• It is always best to buy organic vegetables that have not been treated with pesticides, fertilizers, or preservatives, because they have more nutritive value and contain no toxins. On the other hand, it's better to eat mass-produced vegetables than no vegetables at all.

• You should also try to obtain organically grown plants for your herbal remedies, as well as lemons, onions, honey, etc.

• Always use honey to sweeten infusions and decoctions instead of sugar, because honey is rich in minerals and Vitamins A, C, and E.

• B complex vitamins are destroyed by alcohol.

﹌ The Vitamins

Here's a list that will tell you everything you need to know about vitamins, including what they're good for, daily requirements, and where to find them.

Vitamin A (in the form of pro-vitamin A, which is transformed into Vitamin A by the liver). Benefits growth, eyes, skin, pregnant and breast-feeding women; accelerates healing.

Daily requirement: 1.5 mg

Natural sources: Beets, wheat, chard, raw carrot, celery, cherry, cabbage, cauliflower, squash, watercress, endive, spinach, virgin vegetable oils, lettuce, corn, mandarins, olive, orange, barley, nettle, sorrel, parsley, green pepper, dandelion, fresh peas, plums, prunes, escarole, tomato, sunflower.

B-Complex Vitamins (also see phosphorus). Benefit hair and skin.

Daily requirement: 1.5 mg.

Natural sources: Wheat germ and bran (as well as the germ and bran of other grains), brewer's yeast, whole rice.

Vitamin B1 (thiamin). Benefits digestion; tones the body; combats nerve problems, beriberi, and anemia; helps hair retain its natural color; accelerates healing of certain skin, nervous, and liver disorders.

Daily requirement: 1.5 mg

Natural sources: Garlic, apricots, algae, peanuts, oats, bananas, wheat, wheat germ, blackcurrant, cabbage, dates, dried figs, sprouted wheat, dried beans, lentils, brewer's yeast, melon, hazelnuts, walnuts, barley, oranges, whole grain bread, parsley, dried peas, apples, plums, raisins, lettuce, buckwheat, soya.

Vitamin B2 (riboflavin, also called the longevity vitamin). Stimulates growth in children; prevents cellular oxidation; benefits the eyes, and improves nocturnal vision.

Daily requirement: 2 mg

Natural sources: apricots, beets, sprouted wheat, blackcurrant, cabbage, squash, spinach, wheat and corn flour, wheat germ, brewer's yeast, melon, hazelnuts, oranges, barley, whole grain bread, apples, plums, prunes, raisins, buckwheat, soya.

Vitamin B3 (also called Vitamin PP). Benefits the skin, purifies the blood, prevents oxidation, facilitates digestion, acts as a vasodilator, and improves liver functions.

Daily requirement: 20 mg

Natural sources: whole grains, spinach, whole wheat flour, soya flour, fruits in general, wheat germ, string beans, yeast, molasses, sweet peas, brown rice, barley.

Vitamin B5 (pantothenic acid). Benefits glandular functions and retards the graying of hair.

Daily requirement: 1.5 mg

Natural sources: main sources include royal jelly, wheat germ, brewer's yeast, and pollen; other sources include soya, wheat and rice bran, tomatoes, sunflower seeds, and corn.

Vitamin B10. Necessary for the assimilation of Vitamin L1.

Daily requirement: 20 mg

Natural sources: bananas, grains, mushrooms, cabbage, cauliflower, brewer's yeast, rice bran.

Vitamin B12. Necessary for the formation of red blood cells; combats liver and nerve disorders, migraines, skin problems and anemia (with Vitamin L1).

Daily requirement: 2 mg

Natural sources: algae, brewer's yeast, pollen.

Biotin. Prevents anemia, benefits the skin, improves intellectual functions, and prevents aging.

Daily requirement: 20 mg

Natural sources: banana, wheat, mushrooms, spinach, green beans, brewer's yeast (an excellent source), corn, pollen, potatoes, whole grain rice, tomatoes.

Folic Acid. Promotes growth and the formation of amino acids (a component of proteins).

Daily requirement: 15 mg

Natural sources: asparagus, carrots, spinach, wheat germ.

Inositol. Prevents anemia, accelerates growth, benefits the hair and helps metabolize fats.

Daily requirement: 20 mg

Natural sources: wheat, spinach, royal jelly, brewer's yeast, soya.

Vitamin C (ascorbic acid). Stimulates regeneration of conjunctive tissue, blood vessels, cartilage (teeth and bones), and red blood cells; helps eliminate toxins; prevents fatigue; tones and calms the organism.

Daily requirement: 75 mg (more for smokers and persons suffering from an infection)

Natural sources: garlic, cranberries, artichoke, asparagus, eggplant, beets, chard, blackcurrants, celery, chervil, cherries, chestnuts, chicory, cabbage, brussels sprouts, cauliflower, red cabbage, chives, lemons, cucumber, strawberries, raspberries, guava, grenadine, gooseberries, green beans, kiwi, lettuce, mandarins, mango, melon, myrtle, turnip, hazelnuts, onion, oranges, nettle, grapefruit, parsnip, watermelon, sweet peas, apples, potatoes, plums, radish, horseradish, fresh grapes, rhubarb, rutabaga, escarole, soya, tomatoes, Jerusalem artichokes.

Vitamin D (sunlight is essential for the production of Vitamin D in the body). Regulates metabolism; necessary for the assimilation of calcium; prevents rickets.

Daily requirement: 0.25 mg

Natural sources: algae, almonds, pineapple, oats, soya, sunflower seeds.

Vitamin E (alpha tocopherol). Benefits genital organs, improves fertility and sexuality in general.

Daily requirement: 20 mg

Natural sources: algae, wheat germ, cabbage, watercress, peanut oil, virgin olive oil, soya oil, wheat germ, corn germ, lettuce, walnuts, whole wheat bread, buckwheat, soya.

Vitamin F (linoleic acid). Helps metabolize fats, benefits the skin.

Daily requirement: not specified

Natural sources: asparagus; spinach; unrefined peanut, soya and linseed oil; sweet peas; soya.

Vitamin G (also called Vitamin B6 or pyridoxin). Regulates nervous system and brain functions; promotes better sleep.

Daily requirement: 2 mg

Natural sources: algae; fresh almonds and peanuts; wheat germ; cabbage; watercress; corn germ; virgin peanut, palm and soya oil; lettuce; walnuts; whole wheat bread.

Vitamin J (choline chlorhydrate).

Daily requirement: 20 mg

Natural sources: beets, lemon, liver, brewer's yeast, dandelion.

Vitamin K Necessary for the coagulation of blood.

Daily requirement: 4 mg

Natural sources: algae, oats, cabbage, spinach, strawberries, brewer's yeast, alfalfa sprouts, soya, tomatoes.

Vitamin P (rutin). Protects the internal walls of blood vessels, maintains balanced blood pressure.

Daily requirement: 40 mg

Natural sources: lettuce, pansy leaves, buckwheat.

❧ Minerals

Minerals regulate bodily functions, keep the nervous system healthy, promote better assimilation of nutrients, and regenerate the blood. Important minerals include calcium, copper, iron, magnesium, and silica.

Calcium promotes the formation of collagen, which prevents wrinkles and keeps the skin supple. It is also a natural sedative. Combined with phosphorus it ensures proper skeletal growth and good teeth. Some experts claim this mineral plays a major role in preventing cancer.

Daily requirement: 880 mg

Natural sources: apricots, pineapple, almonds, oats, carrots, blackcurrants, cherries, cabbage, chive, watercress, spinach, corn, blackberries, walnut, onion, barley, sweet peas, dandelion, rice, semolina, soya, tomatoes.

Medicinal plants: Chamomile, Nettle, Sorrel, Queen of the Meadow

Iron is an essential component of blood. It regenerates red blood cells and is also necessary for liver functions. Iron is an essential nutrient, especially for children and pregnant women.

Daily requirement: 0.0016 mg

Natural sources: apricot, pineapple, asparagus, oats, bananas, wheat, celery, spinach, raspberry, lentils, walnuts, oranges, barley, nettle, parsley, leek, potato, rice, tomato.

Medicinal plants: Mullein, Raspberry, Nettle, Water Dock, Parsley, Queen of the Meadow

Copper is necessary for the assimilation of iron. A lack of copper results in prematurely gray hair, and nervous and cardiac problems.

Daily requirement: 2 mg

Natural sources: apricot, pineapple, blackcurrant, chestnut, dates, figs, strawberries, raspberries, walnuts, oranges, sweet peas, parsley.

Medicinal plants: Burdock, Watercress, Kelp, Yarrow, Nettle, Parsley

Iodine is indispensable for the proper functioning of phagocyte cells that destroy microbes and eliminate waste. It is also important for maintaining proper endocrine functions (including thyroid, pituitary, testicle and ovarian functions).

Daily requirement: 100 micrograms

Natural sources: pineapple, artichoke, beets, mushrooms, watercress, spinach, onion.

Medicinal plants: Garlic, Kelp

Magnesium protects the nervous system and acts as a natural sedative. It also plays an important role in preventing cancer. A normal diet should provide you with your daily magnesium requirement.

Daily requirement: 200 mg

Natural sources: bananas, wheat, carrots, red cabbage, onion, oranges, dandelion, rice, rye, tomatoes.

Medicinal plants: Kelp, Peppermint, Walnut, Queen of the Meadow

Phosphorus is essential for assimilating B complex vitamins, which are in turn essential for maintaining proper organic functions. Combined with lecithin, this mineral also helps dissolve fats.

Daily requirement: 5 grams

Natural sources: apricot, almonds, wheat, carrots, lemon, corn, hazelnut, orange, onion, potatoes, sweet peas, dandelion, soya, tomatoes.

Medicinal plants: Garlic, Mullein, Caraway, Sweet Flag, Licorice, Queen of the Meadow, Marigold

Silica helps keep the skin firm and improves vision.

Daily requirement: 2 mg

Natural sources: nettle, dandelion.

Medicinal plants: Comfrey, Lungwort, Horsetail

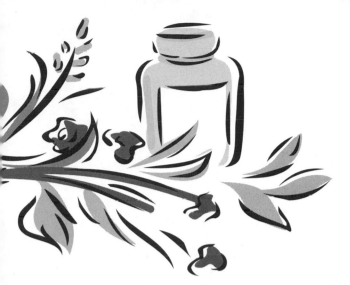

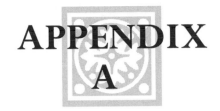

Depurative Remedy

Use 1/3 oz of each of the following ingredients: powdered aloe vera, angelica root, zedoary (round turmeric), rhubarb root, Chinese camphor, senna leaves, manna, Venetian theriaque, and saffron; also use a pinch of myrrh and milk thistle. Mix all these ingredients together in a large glass container and cover with 1-1/2 quarts of good quality 40 proof fruit alcohol. Place the container in direct sunlight or near some other heat source for 15 days. Make sure to agitate the mixture at least once a day. Store in your refrigerator in a tightly sealed container.

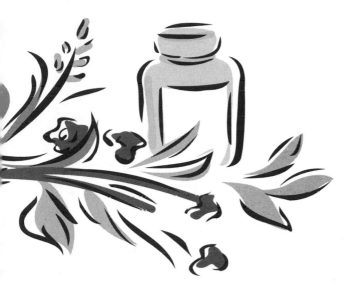

Hypotoxic Diet

This diet is recommended for a large number of disorders, and is designed to eliminate harmful substances and calm the nervous system. You should drink lots of spring water with a low mineral content, and avoid all the foods listed below.

a) **Meat:** fat meat, organ meat, lamb, goat, ham, wild game (especially pheasant), sweetbread, tripe, smoked meats, brain, liver, kidney, poultry, lard.

b) **Meat derivatives**: greasy broth, meat stew, processed meats (except lean ham), canned meat, liver paté, sausages, meat sauce.

c) **Fish:** anchovies, caviar, canned fish or seafood, herring, shellfish, mollusks (except oysters), fat fish, sardines.

d) **Vegetables:** mushrooms, cauliflower, spinach, string beans, rhubarb, asparagus.

e) **Condiments:** spices like pimento, pepper, mustard, vinegar.

f) **Alcohol:** digestives, aperitifs, strong beer, heavy red wine (Bourgogne, port) and champagne.

g) **Other foods to avoid:** all excess fats, greasy or fried foods, mayonnaise, greasy sauces, pastry, fermented cheeses (blue, brie, Roquefort, etc.), chocolate, cacao, oleaginous fruit, strong tea or coffee, eggs (if the disorder is related to a liver problem, chronic nephritis or high blood pressure), and soft white bread.

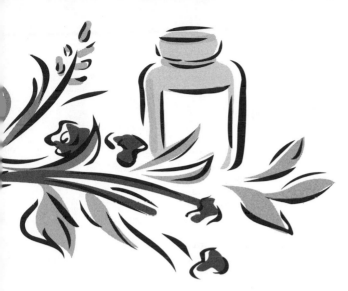

Index